Social Sadomasochism

Social Sadomasochism

HOW EMOTIONAL DOMINANCE AND SUBMISSION AFFECT PEOPLE'S LIVES

Martin Kantor, MD

PRAEGER®

An Imprint of ABC-CLIO, LLC
Santa Barbara, California • Denver, Colorado

Library of Congress Cataloging in Publication Control Number: 2019021040

ISBN: 978-1-4408-6320-2 (print)
978-1-4408-6321-9 (ebook)

23 22 21 20 19 1 2 3 4 5

This book is also available as an eBook.

Praeger
An Imprint of ABC-CLIO, LLC

ABC-CLIO, LLC
147 Castilian Drive
Santa Barbara, California 93117
www.abc-clio.com

This book is printed on acid-free paper ♾

Manufactured in the United States of America

Dedicated to Michael

Contents

Introduction

A Summary

Many authors, Blum among them, have pondered the personal aspects of sadomasochism, specifically, the reasons for (causality of) individual sadomasochism—that is, the role that sadomasochism plays in personal emotional dysfunction. They have mostly concluded that according to Holtzman and Kulish quoting Blum, masochism is simply "consciously or unconsciously seeking pain, suffering, and humiliation."[1] But still poorly understood/mainly ignored is the heart of that matter: why would someone be altruistic (self-sacrificial) if that meant failing to act in a selfish, that is, self-protective, manner? Why would anyone act in a hurtful way to oneself if he or she sensibly realized that the way to nirvana consisted of at least appearing to be overly generous and giving to others? Why would anyone turn his or her daily life into an exercise of self-defeat? Why would anyone be the principle pinion of like-minded groups of men and women out to collectively harm themselves, hurt the opposition, or do both at the same time so that nobody thrives yet no one escapes?

I understand how some groups want to relieve the suffering of (other) oppressed groups, a noble aim. But what is hard to fathom is why these groups themselves become antisocial organizations breaking our society apart in the process of seeming to put it together, as if reducing the active suffering (of others) should be their fundamental/real objective, but see helping themselves thrive as forbidden because doing so is unhealthy and amoral, especially if it involves opposing other groups currently seeking some of the fame and all of the power. But this is the reality. Self-harm and being sadistic to others nevertheless affects the highest levels of society: from staff in the White House on down to leaders of our households and from the top gun to the ordinary rifleman out to cripple our own houses and spreading to the workplace, with ourselves beholden to bosses with whom we spend a third or so of our lives, wasting our time and money as we deliberately, almost defiantly, even fiendishly, let them impinge on our well-being/sensibilities, ruin our finances, disrupt our love relationships, and stifle our potential creativity. We work hard for others, only to have them work as hard against us to cancel the good with the bad, the hope with the despair, the mirth with the sorrow—to, in other words, themselves actually make the world not a lovely place to live in but a dysfunctional operation forcing those who set out to make things better to instead become functionless, with pain and suffering the default, hate the primary motivation, and spite the sung or unsung mantra.

Psychodynamically, cognitively, interpersonally, sexually, and morally as well as socioeconomically, it seems difficult to impossible to fathom why individuals and groups of individuals work singly or in concert with self-defeat, with failure being their most cherished of goals, the disruption of their lives the happiest of their dreams, wiping that smile off the faces of others, the joyous emoji, the heart of their intentions, as they create adversaries out of people who were previously their friends but can now never again become their allies. Why is so much we see on a day-to-day basis of such a self-destructive nature, seemingly passively originating in experienced "not my fault" disappointments in life but in fact actively constructed out of spite and engineered out of rage, all to create suffering as one's objective, with certain pleasures forbidden even to the healthy, moral, well-functioning individual and instead belonging only to a fantastic few, a subgroup of unhealthy self-flagellators who brag to the world using their private richly festooned banners of "see how I suffer" as a way to say "stay away from me and don't try to live my life for me, or I will make you suffer in kind," as when they are seemingly concerned for the well-being of all, they get too powerful, and bring the whole country down on its knees to gratify some fond secret wish of their own? Can't we ever see the foolishness of how being hurtful these ways swallows itself up in its own waste: energy depleted, functionality disrobed, and even our own continued existence threatened just to make some questionable philosophical point as we simultaneously, like Cassandra, the philosopher of doom, gleefully preside over, even happily cause, the deplorable destruction of everything around us that is good in the guise of enhancing the pleasure we get out of what for some, and in some ways even for all, are immensely pleasurable surroundings—as there we sit, situated at the edge of a verdant cliff, just waiting and hoping for the clouds to come by and the earth to rumble and to throw us over the edge into the widespread orbit of disgrace and pain that lies at the bottom of a pit of doom, one we yearn to meet head-on, as a way to cripple ourselves so that we can no longer do our best but remain able to only function at our possible imaginable worst?

Clearly, what we are dealing with is the self-defeating character. But due in part to the various complexities associated with this character (neurosis), few observers have successfully addressed (and not uncovered convincingly the answer to) the question of how to understand such a person and how understanding him and her and the sadomasochism that rules over all concerned can tell us at least something about the answers to some of the most pressing questions about these individuals, people who seem unable to work through the self-defeating tendencies so many people take along with them in their ventures throughout life and to their graves. First as children, then as adolescents, and then as adults with the child within (psychologically) following right along, we have what Millon calls (in his discussion of masochism) that person "characterized by self-criticism, a querulous disposition, and a habit of tormenting both self and others." As Millon continues, "such a person, a masochist, is, however, in a terrible bind. Love and affection are sought but result in pain; by making [oneself] unlovable, masochists avoid some pain but, as a consequence, prevent themselves from achieving the love they desire."[2]

Indeed, most of those who have studied the problem seem not only to have stopped short of enlightenment but also to have drawn specific conclusions that seem more on the mark than they actually are. In the process of missing the bull's-eye, they narrowly conclude that individual sadomasochism is the product of social sadomasochism—that is, individuals pick up and act on the premise that society makes them what they are, and it is cruel societies that breed cruel people. This, though a part truth, is an overgrown oversimplification. To me, the real and more serious problem is that cruel people, sensing that like breeds like, flock together to form cohorts whereby each member is or is soon to become sadomasochistic, and it is their affinity toward each other that leads to the formation of groups valuing cruelty above all, pockets of people who, having joined hands, become not only hateful to each other but also proselytizers of cruelty all around, setting themselves off from other groups they are surrounded by, themselves having come together to exclude or even to despise other bands of men and women with whom they refuse to come into or stay in prolonged generative contact. I am speaking not only of the physical torturer but also of the teacher who knows it all, so you can't tell him or her anything, or of the friend who takes every question as an attack, so it's not "do you ask just because you want to know?" but "you have no respect for me and are trying to tell me who I am and how to live my life."

Clearly, then, a goal of a book on sadomasochism must be to attempt to shed a brighter light on the self-defeating character, the personal characteristic (trait) and the character (neurosis), behaviors that all of us display at various times and in various ways in all of our lives and thus a problem that to some respect we all have and must identify and correct if we are to remedy the difficulty as it exists both in the individual and in the society in which he or she lives. The problem for sadomasochistic individuals, however, is this: each time in most lives of both individuals and sadomasochist groups, one or all make certain that whenever they come to a forked road the termination of which is clearly marked as being a dead end, they are attracted to taking the branch of the roadway that leads to the premature stoppage of positive outcomes just to see what lies beyond. And somehow they sense where they are going in advance, so when seeking pleasure and success they often seem instead to be inadvertently seeking unpleasure and failure by doing the exact opposite of what they are warned in advance not to do. Where the pleasure principle might guide them, turning tragedy into comedy, they go exactly the other way around and are left not with pleasure but with pain of a widespread and sometimes excruciating nature.

In this book, I try to evolve therapeutic interventions that can help remedy individual, group, and social sadomasochistic dysfunction. Material in this regard is presented after being researched in the literature, and new formulations are made based on my having worked therapeutically with both child and adult sadomasochists; thus, suggestions as to description, causality, and therapy are not mine alone (and therefore are not based strictly on my personal clinical experience as a psychiatrist) but also emanate out of my observations of humanity and as a social human from living with these unfortunate problems, mine and others, on a day-to-day basis.

A special mystery of sadomasochistic life is that some people seek dissatisfaction as the royal road to satisfaction and the reverse, affiliating themselves with what appear to be moral paradoxes, such as "Why do we have the need to deliberately torture ourselves with disturbing thoughts or purposively torture ourselves with doomed visual and cognitive scenarios?," based on the belief that so much of what we see on a day-to-day basis is of such a self-destructive nature, seemingly originating in passively experienced "not my fault" terrible events beyond our control, when in fact what happens to us is actively constructed not out of bad luck or is there in our genes, coming out in the form of spite and anger and the allure of disgust, but instead is engineered by the motivation to break our society apart and make attack from within look like spoilage from without. In the process we mistreat ourselves as if suffering now and later is a product of our helplessness when in fact we are motivated to subject ourselves and our fellow human beings to displeasure, an excess thereof considered to be healthy and an absence thereof considered to be not only morally acceptable but also highly desirable.

A psychoanalytic approach in an attempt to answer why sadomasochists do this to themselves and others views the problem from the following aspects: the id, or unconscious; the superego, or conscience; the ego ideal, or one's motivations and goals in life; and the ego, which is the organizing integrating aspects of the psyche that attempt to make compromises between these often sometimes disparate forces in one's emotional life, all of which press to be in charge while remaining vague as to which ought to be dominant and how they should mesh with one another. Figuratively, speaking in the vernacular, such people tell themselves that this world has people in it at the ready to "eat each other up alive" (oral sadomasochism), "sully the other" (anal sadomasochism), extract "an eye for an eye" (phallic sadomasochism), and set as their goals seeking the likes of failure rather than success, self-punishment rather than admirable achievement, and at least formulate goals for themselves that reflect how they deliberately, if unconsciously, are acting beneath their potential capacities and below their abilities to do what is right and all the right things.

In my attempts to try to explain sadomasochism I use vernacular words and phrases, often those used by the sadomasochists themselves. Thus, I quote Agatha Christie, who says in her book *Appointment with Death,* "You think old Mrs. Boyton is a kind of sadist? I am almost sure of it. I think she rejoices in the infliction of pain—mental pain, mind you, not physical. That is very much rarer and very much more difficult to deal with. She likes to have control of other human beings and she likes to make them suffer."[3]

Such vernacular formulations go, as many psychiatrists have said, "right to the id" or, using a non-Freudian term, "straight to the heart of the matter," doing so in my opinion more directly than some of the complex psychoanalytic formulations that exist in what literature there is about sadomasochism. An emphasis on the preoedipal fixation of the sadomasochist, however accurate it may be, might at first seem incisive but turn out to not actually be a helpful contribution to meaningful knowledge of the process. An honest academic (but hard to understand/apply) discussion of the regressive (infantile) nature of sadomasochistic dyads is not too useful for the everyday clinician struggling with patients whose creativity consists of ways to harm themselves and not tell the analyst that is what they are up to. And a discussion of how sadomasochists act out their personal introjects with libidinally valued others is perhaps better replaced with information about how sadomasochists are fond of always hurting the ones they love the most. Attempts to answer the questions "What is sadomasochism, a self-defeating personality disorder?," "Where and how does it arise?," and "How can we, after identifying it, clinically and socially improve society so that we live as nonsadomasochists who usefully and positively resort to commonsense solutions to everyday problems?" effectively employ methods that are at best semi-Freudian. With this in mind, it may be helpful to resort to the hearty use of analogy, though this is not fundamentally scientific and is indeed anti-Freudian. Thus, quoting Agatha Christie again, in her book *The Moving Finger*[4] she might have been speaking of sadomasochism when she wrote about that "black inward unhappiness—like a septic arm physically, all black and swollen. If you could cut it and let the poison out, it would flow away harmlessly. Yes, poor soul, poor soul." Analogies such as these soon break down, but up to a point this helps us understand why somebody would want to work at cross-purposes to himself or herself and would find the biblical suggestion to "love thy neighbor" if not laughable, then in today's neighborhoods, at least according to the individual's own personality structure, unproductive, inadvisable, and practically speaking indefensible.

Attempting to understand sadomasochism via reference to fiction (and nonfiction) can be equally helpful for revealing crucial aspects of sadomasochism. Reading the well-known story about the oral sadomasochism of the human vampire bat teaches us something and is thrilling in addition to being revealing, as are the many stories in the Bible and in mythology that deal with premature and untimely ends of heroic characters (such as the horrific demise of poor John the Baptist who instead of fighting back underwent a sadistic "castration" at the hands of the equally sadistic King Herod, enabling the fearsome sadomasochistic wishes of the terrible Salome to come to fruition). The 12 trials of Hercules and Delilah's shearing of Sampson's locks, sapping his strength, are stories of heroes who do more penance in a day than almost any imaginable individual or group collectively does in an entire lifetime, and in at least Salome's case, her terrible end may reveal how she was an ultimate masochist at heart (doing her Dance of Death).

My book tells the familiar story of the need of an individual or a group to identify a rival and abusively show him or her up—someone to fight with or conquer not as an inspirational climax in the form of an outburst of camaraderie, equality, and the final joy of love but rather as the tale of the individual breakups of a "love affair," the boss firing one of his or her best workers, or the political group out not to challenge a rival group's policy/philosophy for good reason but instead to dismember a rival group's potentially finest intellectual and worldly achievements. We tell the all-too-familiar story of becoming a cropper of destruction by one's own hand as the sadistic boomerang turns into the ultimate masochistic weapon, harming the one who threw it into the air in the first place only to experience surprise at where exactly it fell to Earth.

PART 1

Recognizing the Elements

1

Introduction

An Overview

THEORIES OF MASOCHISM

Authors agree with Glick and Meyers that "[masochism] involve[s] an obligatory connection between pain and pleasure [which is] self-motivated, [and] self-destructive."[1] They note that Krafft-Ebing defined masochism as "the wish to suffer pain and be subjected to force, the idea of being completely and unconditionally subject to the will of a person of the opposite sex; of being treated by this person, as by a master, humiliated, and abused."[2] Berliner proposed that masochism means "loving a person who gives hate and ill treatment,"[3] and Brenner said that "the essence of masochism appears to consist in an intimate relationship between pleasure and pain. There is a seeking of unpleasure by which is meant physical or mental pain.[4] Cooper saw masochism as a "variety of pleasurable goals or gratifications arising at all levels of psychic development."[5]

MASOCHISM AND ITS VARIOUS CAUSAL THEORIES

The Literature

The earliest formulations about the nature of masochism saw it as a defense, that is, as a way of dealing with anxiety; later formulations emphasized object relations theory, that is, the place that masochism and sadomasochism take in relationships. Viewing sadomasochism much like passive-aggression as a dyadic disorder, they note that the presence of another person is required to fit the bill.

Freud (1915) originally stressed that sadism was "primary, based on the aggressive drive to master, and masochism represented redirecting the aggression onto the self and changing the mode from active to passive." The masochist achieves gratification by identifying with the sadist in the act. Freud also emphasized "the defensive nature of masochism, not simply or exclusively its instinctual nature." His formulation reflects the evolving importance of the superego, which provokes a sense of guilt for sexual and aggressive drives. In moral masochism the suffering itself is "all that matters."[6] Guilt can be a distraction or can represent a need for punishment. Also, guilt is a preliminary to retribution, making masochism instinctual and defensive. As derived from the establishment of the superego and the wish to submit to the father and as a defense against castration danger, masochism is ultimately passive and feminine.

According to Horney, the masochist has established "the strategic value of suffering to defend against the fears associated with feelings of intrinsic weakness. Though suffering is painful, abandoning oneself to excessive suffering may serve as an opiate against pain."[7] Aggression is seen as far more impotent or basic in masochism than sexuality.

Markman noted that overall "masochism protects the patient from overwhelming anxiety in facing separateness and dependency on an object outside the self."[8]

As Sugarman says, "in general my experience . . . with masochistic psychopathology is that aggression, far more than sexuality, is the drive being managed and expressed through the masochistic symptom or character trait."[9]

And Margolis finds masochism "organized around sadistic and primitive superego functions,"[10] simultaneously permitting, in a compromise formation, gratification and punishment for forbidden incestuous sexual wishes so that, he says, "masochism in the case of sexual boundary violators and their patients is almost always interwoven with narcissism, superego pathology, and often a desperate neediness, all of which may be embedded in individuals who have many strengths, talents and virtues."

Later observers stress how critical it is to look at the level of the person's object relations in evaluating the quality of masochism. For example, one idea is that a masochistic relationship is experienced as being better than no relationship at all, that pain must be suffered in order to keep the early object tie, or that such a relationship represents a struggle to take control over the painful loss of early omnipotence or to master and claim victory over calamity and trauma. The masochistic individual, in suffering, may hold on to an inner sense of narcissistic triumph over those who might wish to help her or him.

Crossover theories exist. For example, from a vantage point of self-psychology, masochism is understood as a means of repairing a faulty or fragile self, holding a fragmenting sense of self together in the midst of ongoing dissolution, or regulating (smoothing over) one's feelings. According to object relations theory, masochism may be viewed as the manifestation of identifying with hostile despised parental images.

COVALENCE

Sadomasochism is rarely pure; mostly it presents in association with multiple psychiatric covalent disorders accompanied by nonsadomasochistic features that cause a severe degree of often cumulative and progressive suffering for so many individuals and throughout our society. As a result, sadomasochism presents in a given individual as overlapping diagnostically with other personality disorders, especially depression and paranoia, so that we have not pure sadomasochism but instead mixed personality disorders. In large measure, this is because sadomasochism and other personality disorders utilize many of the same (concealing) defenses meant to be hurtful in the extreme while concealing the motivation of the wish to be thus, sacrificing some freedom of open expression in order to maintain the "confidentiality" of what one is really thinking and feeling. Thus, one patient got my sympathy by telling me the story of how her dog bit a friend on the thumb, emphasizing how the friend was unfairly demanding money from her in compensation. What she left out was that the dog had been biting people for years and that this time the wound got infected and the person bitten had to spend three days in the hospital running up a huge bill, payment of which by the insurance company was by no means assured.

Put another way, each neurotic or psychotic behavior contains a *sadomasochistic* core at its hub, or the possibility likely exists that there is a sadomasochistic basis to all neuroses. As a result, sadomasochism is often hard to tease out from such comorbid disorders with similar defenses as covalent avoidance, where *interpersonal removal* is chosen as the primary hurtful/protective mechanism ("he, not I, destroyed that relationship"); *reaction formation,* where one says and does the opposite of what one means (e.g., using such defeating mechanisms of irony as killing with kindness, as typified by oily overconcern for the fate of others when one is in fact not truly concerned at all about what happens to them, only hoping to hear tragedy); regression, becoming childlike to disavow adult responsibility by, say, citing so-called can't-be-helped developmental fixation as being at the root of all adult misbehavior and to explain the origin of some evil they are doing as "not me but my preoedipal conflicts"; rationalization, as when intellectual spin is used to justify emotional action and reaction such as in the citing of social pressures/approval (seeking political correctness), thereby excusing one's sadomasochism under the guise of its fitting in with some in-group to which one belongs, though the political correctness here happens to only be of a theoretical nature; compromise formation, whereby two opposing ideas are forged into one that expresses both while emphasizing neither, leaving behind a communicative pastiche that is open to more than one interpretation; denial, directed to being able to sadistically proclaim one's innocence by developing a "not me, not ever" stance in regard to one's past, present, and likely future beliefs and actions, thus proving oneself beyond reproach no matter how hard another tries to affix the blame on an in-fact guilty party; and omission, such as when a patient first said she was going to commit suicide by going off her medications but failed to report that by now she had arranged an assisted suicide in a state that permitted this for some patients who wished not to live a long time with an illness that may have ultimately turned out to be chronic, not, as she averred, acute.

Common defense mechanisms also include *turning around on the self,* also characteristic of depression, and *selective abstraction,* also characteristic of psychopathy, where the intent is to buffalo others by eliminating information that goes contrary to a central point one wants to make regardless of the truth and validity of the whole story, here told by omitting/avoiding certain valid aspects of the truth in order to selectively refer to only one element or a few insignificant minor (though meaningful) valid elements of the reality, not as a revelation but as a concealment.

Grandiosity—bragging about one's attributes to people who might not want to hear about them—can be a defense against low self-esteem. Bragging about taking responsibility for oneself often takes the form of sadomasochistic behavior along the lines of "you see, don't you? I am in touch with myself in this way" and "don't need anyone else's help." A fear of being inadequate leads to *hyperadequacy behaviors* as a contrast. *Distracting oneself* involves performing diverting distracting masochistic acts, such as taking lessons to play an instrument one will never play or wasting money one needs for vocational school.

A *fear of being independent* leads one to play the sick role and a fear of being sick, leading to hyperhealthy behaviors that take the form of extremes of hurtful independence (e.g., not taking care of oneself to stay alive for someone who loves you and to die on that someone out of spite).

A forbidden wish to drive others away leads to the masochism of avoidant personality disorder (AVPD). Comorbid fears of intimacy and closeness, coupled with a wish to be autonomous and independent, are present in avoidant sadomasochistic behaviors, where the prevailing goal—to antagonize others with masochism—is in fact distancing behavior that can be a sadistic form of removal. Many want to have their needs met without having to ask for others to do so, part of the spiteful wish to be passively loved unconditionally and without having to beg for it on the one hand and without being ambushed by love on the other hand.

To explain the wordless nature of some sadomasochistic activity, it might be that the core defenses are action-level defenses coming earlier in development before one has achieved a capacity to symbolize (so that one has to inquire whether the person cannot express his or her feelings in words, because the key injury occurred so early in life).

Sexual and anger restraints of a defensive nature play a significant role in the psychogenesis of disorders other than hysteria and passive-aggression. Because covert sexuality and anger are found to be characteristic of a number of diverse disorders, the mere presence of hidden anger and other emotions alone does not automatically equate with the diagnosis of passive-aggression, sadomasochistic personality disorder, or any other specific disorder. Also, while all sadomasochists hold back their anger in some way, not all hold back their emotions in the same way, so different sadomasochists express their sexuality and anger in different ways; that is, they do so by the use of different emotional styles consisting of different compromises (defenses) against anger.

To some extent, the nature and the seriousness of any example of sadomasochism varies with the degree to which one is emotionally overburdened and how one deals with that: projecting accounting for paranoia, introjection accounting for depression, and so on.

It is also true that whatever category they fall into, sadomasochists treat themselves in much the same way they treat others. Thus, sadomasochism is sometimes mainly an alloplastic disorder (where others get hurt) *or* one that is autoplastic (where one suffers only oneself). That is, patients who express anger at others are ultimately often as sadomasochistic as they are sadistic or masochistic.

Whether alloplastic or autoplastic, while the means and object of one's emotions of anger and sexual expression differ from case to case, some similarities of purpose and method are retained in all or almost all cases. To illustrate, many sadomasochists effectively express anger at themselves and others by depriving themselves of the various satisfactory methods of relational or impersonal gratification. This is illustrated by a patient who was a main object of his own anger. Since he felt guilty about having made too much money, he appeased his unreasonable conscience, placating his sense of guilt by sadomasochistically taking arduous subway trips instead of going to work by a cab, which he could easily afford to hire. Of course, this being another one of his prime purposes, he also involved other people simultaneously in his problem. In his case the public transportation in town was so bad that when he relied on it he could always expect to be late for work, in that way not only inconveniencing himself but also annoying his coworkers and simultaneously being especially troubling to his boss.

Some sadomasochists go contrary to the classic model and express themselves (e.g., their anger) directly. This might happen when what Benjamin calls an "inside ball of anger" explodes as defenses relative to "guilty anger and blame issues" break down and do so with a great impact on relationships.[11] Here the mechanisms of indirect expression of anger become invalidated; as subtle defiance no longer pertains and as defenses break down, the patient gives way to rage. This overt rage, which may be verbalized or with difficulty controlled by transformative acting out, is more likely than oblique anger to be associated with specific external provocation. The rage can also occur seemingly spontaneously and take the form of verbalized temper tantrums that are essentially releases, sometimes pleasurable, of a general sense of pent-up aggression. If the object of the angry behavior retaliates in kind so much the better, for now the victim's response is used to go back and justify the initial attack (diminishing the patient's current guilt), and in any case the result is a set-to that subsequently affords the patient the fullest scope for expression of what anger remains.

In many instances patients express and control their anger, simultaneously leading to seething. Seething is one form of the many *sadistic anger styles* that characterize one of the different types of sadomasochistic expression of anger.

RECLASSIFICATION OF SADOMASOCHISM

Sadomasochism is not the only personality disorder with self-defeating features. Paranoid personality disorder is a leader among the others—think of the unduly suspicious tyrant who attacks an innocent on the subway platform, only to be jumped and beaten up by a group of strangers trying to rescue the victim. But sadomasochism is one of the more complex psychological problems, one with widespread and multiple clinical features and psychodynamic causes, the latter of which (causes) are overdetermined, as this disorder originates developmentally in different significant psychological levels of growth and development, therefore serving various functions and creating various problems as the baby, starting with day one of having been born, grows older and often but not necessarily wiser and when older retains and retraces various ontological and phylogenetic earlier stages of his or her life, a study of which contributes in depth to our understanding of the long-held secrets of the pleasure in the pain of the adult sadomasochist. This helps explain why those seriously wounded (psychologically or physically) in the past, anyone with a major injury, who might want to repeat the familiar would and could seek dissatisfaction as the royal road to satisfaction and enjoy the pain and suffering of another person, often one who is him or herself innocent and has done no one any harm whatsoever.

We may profitably see sadomasochism as a derivative disorder, a complication associated with this final period (the genital stage) of development and thought. So, should we reclassify our familiar disorders such as passive-aggressive personality disorder, where anger is expressed indirectly as one form of, or as the mother of, sadomasochism? What is the relationship between obsessive-compulsive personality disorder (OCPD) or drug addiction and sadomasochism? Many disorders bear a relationship to or contain a component of self-defeat and torturing others. And perhaps so do all, since it is the rare emotional disorder where both others and oneself are not made to suffer. (The chapter on comorbid disorders discusses this further.)

Should we completely reclassify sadomasochism to the more well-known disorder of which it is a part (i.e., narcissistic personality disorder), where lack of empathy is the familiar hurtful focus, or to passive-aggressive personality disorder and call anger expressed indirectly "sadomasochistic"? Since so many disorders bear a relationship to or contain a component of sadomasochism, does the close relationship between other disorders such as narcissism, OCPD, and drug addiction even warrant our not seeing sadomasochism as a separate disorder, even one that hardly exists in its own right?

CAUSALITY: DIFFERENT PATHS TO SELF-DEFEAT

Many different ways to sadomasochism exist for a child to grow up to become a self-destructive adult. There are direct and indirect causal pathways for developing the bad habits of constant self-recrimination and hurtfulness to self/others and becoming a nasty person whom few people, if anyone, want to deal with. Parenthetically, hurtful venues can serve as substitutes one for the other, as cutting oneself substitutes for head banging or breath holding. Many of these developmental pathways are notable for retracing introjects of our parents' attitudinal positions, the ones they routinely assumed while bringing us up. Some of these are controversial pathways such as the ones about spanking and setting limits and other behaviors that are neither widely accepted nor generally advocated. Why can cutting oneself be chosen over other methods of atonement? The nature (the content) and severity (intensity) of guilt is one of the distinctive building blocks here; mild guilt is likely to produce the mostly symbolic head banging or breath holding, whereas more severe guilt is likely to produce the more destructive and relatively overlooked cutting of one's arms, laddering slices from the wrist up to the shoulder, making certain that others who have a right to be concerned get the point about the patient's relationship to himself or herself as well as to family and friends.

Sadomasochism helps explain self-destructiveness, but what is it that explains sadomasochism? Is it a primary problem or disorder, inborn or acquired? Is it chosen by, or for, the individual? Is sadomasochism itself a fundamental stance or one that is derivative of something else, something more basic, such as a psychological spinoff of a biological survival mechanism (ego-defense), related, for example, to hunger, so that there is the need to maintain one's nutrition or die so one doesn't give up even if self-punishment requires cruel abuse using the different rules of self-destruction that incontrovertibly govern the food chain to ensure that we eat and the other laws of the jungle that help keep us from being nutritionally deprived or otherwise physically endangered, however much that in turn assures us that something or someone else will suffer that very destruction or even death as a result of our behavior?

DEVELOPMENT

Various theories of the development of sadomasochism exist; they are not so different one from the other, which means that there are very few distinctive ones.

Aggression first experienced toward the self can soon become experienced toward another, that is, as object-directed. The masochist clings to the regressive and destructive parent-child relationship. According to Asch, "severe separation anxiety and the unwillingness to give up an exclusive but destructive attachment is similar to the dynamic of many battered children and their relationship with the battering mother."[12]

Identification with someone, generally a parent who served as a model of masochism in the person's childhood, is an important causal factor. Other gratifications include maintenance of object relations or self-definition or self-esteem enhancement. Exhibitionistic drives prevail, and the pleasures of self-pity surmount the pleasures of success.

As the baby grows older he or she passes through a number of stages, consecutively or mostly simultaneously. These notably include oral, anal, and phallic/genital developmental phases. In this progression he or she has to learn/be taught/evolve ways to observe, understand, and master the conflicts and tensions associated with each phase—infantile actions and interactions ruled over by the mother/father—and to deal both in actuality and symbolically by properly handling issues having to do with the child's dependency, anality, and phallic/oedipal events, forming a paramount tangle of interactive tissues all of which predictably elicit strong counterresponses on the part of others, including the parents, involved in the child's care as well as subsequently on the part of the child him or herself. The inability to work through resultant conflicts in a meaningful way can and likely will present the toddler with insurmountable challenges to his or her equilibrium that when left unregulated and untreated, should treatment be necessary, likely leave aftereffects that show up as pathology in the adult, possibly in the adult's preference for perverse nonsexual and sexual expressions involving hurtfulness about dependency (issues of leaving and being left), control (issues of who is going to have whose way), and competition issues (figuratively, who is the lord of this manor). Depending on the baby's constitution and the parental reaction (especially involving issues of guilt and shame, innate or induced), responses are laid down that at first seem benign, only to develop sotto voce and reappear in the adult in the form of often serious sadomasochistic positional preferences such as the following:

In the nonsexual realm of orality, issues of leaving and being left, unreliability (being someone you cannot count on), and not being forthcoming to one's family and friends.

In the sexual realm of orality, varieties of compulsive sexuality.

In the nonsexual realm of anality, issues of control of others, not being clean and neat in one's appearance, and being disorganized (out of control) in one's behavior.

In the sexual realm of anality, smearing, coprophagia, osphresiolagnia, coprophilia, and coprolalia (all ways of pathologically playing with feces) and, with preoccupations with feces, develop over concern about sex being dirty.

In the nonsexual realm of phallic matters, concerns about competition/rivalry along with concerns involving power issues—matters about who figuratively is on top, simultaneously, sometimes literally (and sometimes figuratively) as well.

In the sexual realm of phallic matters, problems of urolagnia, premature ejaculation, painful insertion and withdrawal (dyspareunia), premature ejaculation, and being impeded sexually by fear of castration (leading to self-protective distancing).

Put another way, so much of the psychic life of the sadomasochist is based on unconscious reversions to early history, now long consciously forgotten, and painful psychological traumas, now deliberately or semiconsciously disremembered (repressed).

For example, a critic of my books says that I apply the term "patient" indiscriminately, to include those who are not actively under my care but also those who are psychologically ill for any reason and not necessarily under anyone's care, and says that I do so to make it look like I am a very busy doctor with more patients than I can handle. This is of course not my motivation; what is involved is my desire to clearly present analogies and examples of points I am making by using any clinical material (sick people) I find helpful for illustrative purposes to present to the reader in a helpful and clearly illustrative way. But the reality is that I think my rival is competing with me, making it easier for him to do so by putting me down with fake accusations in an accusatory manner.

NORMAL VERSUS ABNORMAL SADOMASOCHISM

Clearly, then, with sadomasochism it is hard to differentiate normal from abnormal. This makes it difficult for us to see if sadomasochism affects us or our elected leaders in the White House on down to the bosses of the workplace where we spend a third or so of our lives, wasting time and money failing to recognize how sadomasochism impinges on our functionality as well as our sensibilities, our finances, our love relationships, and overall our potential creativity. We do not even know how to avoid feeling sheepish/helpless, for as we try to function in a healthy fashion we discover problems we didn't even know we had, as we foolishly rebel against leaders who make sense and just as foolishly submit to those who don't do things that are in our best interests. All of us discover that with sadomasochists we can only win some of the time, for at other times we virtually must be on the losing end of the terror, unconsciously directed to us and/or formed and/or deliberately distributed around us. Here are some basic dilemmas we all have when dealing with the sadomasochistic personality, including that found in ourselves:

Say "yes" to a masochist and we are being sadistic (because a "yes" hurts someone who needs to be deprived by a "no").

Say "no" to a masochist and we are being sadistic (by depriving him or her of something he or she should have and really needs).

Say "yes" to a sadist and we are being sadistic by allowing him or her free rein when it is limit setting that he or she needs, regardless of what he or she seems to want.

Say "no" to a sadist and we are being sadistic (because that "no" hurts him or her via depriving the sadist of what he/she seemingly wants most of all).

Giving advice presents all of us with a dilemma even when advice is asked for. Those trying to intervene with good advice can feel helpless if not dishonest, as the person asked for advice finds that if you don't give it you are being uncooperative; if you do give it you are probably wrong, for at least it's incomplete; and if you stay silent you are likely to be seen as uncooperative or incompetent. Someone asks, "Should I, now that I am getting older, just downsize my living quarters (house) and continue to try to get along by myself staying indoors and having food delivered, or should I go into a senior living arrangement where I might be less lonely but I might also lose my independence?"

One's response to a sadomasochist is akin to holding a glass with water in it up to your eyes and determining if the glass is half full or half empty. Clearly the other person always wins here because one objective of sadomasochism is defeat, of ourselves or of another person, either indirectly by being difficult (e.g., by putting the other person in a double bind) or directly by being hurtful and striking out at someone aware of what we are doing and creating and often suffering for it. Even those who try come up short, pointing out that in the lack of functionality/foolishness of this particular set of interactions on the part of all concerned they can't win either, because they are effectively exposing the overall futility of trying to please someone whose goal is to be displeased and to defeat those who are trying to help (the "masochistic triumph"). Can you imagine my dilemma when a friend asked me to be her medical proxy, then after I agreed to sign told me she was planning to kill herself?

I am sitting in the front seat of the car when a friend sitting in the backseat tells me that come March she is going to stop her blood thinner and die because she no longer wants to live. I am a board-certified psychiatrist with much experience dealing with suicidal patients. I respond with the best advice I know how to give: get help. She tells me to stop trying to run her life for her. This is sadomasochism in action; the self-defeating personality of everyday life marches triumphantly ahead but along the road that clearly says "Dead End."

To stop the countrywide opioid addiction, doctors are prohibited from prescribing oxycodone except under certain limited circumstances. The patient with severe pain is deprived of his or her medicine. He or she turns to the streets to get heroin or turns to large doses of over-the-counter painkillers, harming the liver or the heart.

A man being interviewed for a government job is unfairly attacked on all sides to the point that he bursts into tears. His allies see him as a wonderful, sensitive human being; his enemies see him as too weak to be successful at a job fraught with tension and conflict.

A worker is late for work and finds himself called untrustworthy; he is early for work and finds himself called dependent; he is on time for work and finds himself called obsessional. He discovers that the double bind is a favorite tool of sadomasochists longing to be hurtful.

I cite as another example the man with no source of income other than gifts from his mother. He nevertheless antagonized her over nothing and lost all of his income as a result. My objection and worry was that in reality he had a self-destructive aspect to his nature that disrupted his positive and practically oriented object relationship with his mother. But this was met by the argument that his was a philosophical bent that advised him to strive for something higher on principle than just raiding someone else's bank account. He then quit therapy after averring that he accepted this problem in his personality, telling me he overcame this side of his personality by assuring me that he read that, as Fenichel says, all real mental phenomena in all people are composed of various "mixtures" of qualities.[13] And things were no different for him.

SOCIAL CAUSATIONS

Few have even begun to tackle the role that sadomasochism plays in creating *social* sadomasochistic dysfunction (i.e., why defined groups of individuals and aspects or the whole of what they constitute seem bent to appoint a leader and follow the leader to destruction, their own or that of a rival group, doing so even when alternate approaches to their own problems and methods for problem solving of others (challenging group solutions) are readily available or are available though perhaps with a degree of difficulty that requires expanding the search for healthy adult functioning methods that involve working together to reach a common goal. The results of some elections seem to prove that some sadomasochistic people are better at feeling strongly than they are at thinking correctly.

Clearly the individual is not always alone in being affected by sadomasochism. There is an overlap today between an individual's sadomasochistic personality disorder and group sadomasochistic personality disorder, especially when it involves political activism, one that is striking (e.g., "kick 'em when they are down"). Sadomasochists tend to flock together and form a poorly functioning (but rarely efficient) group, with prohibitions and preferences, aversions and attractions, and viewing things from the perspective of ways that sadomasochism can affect one negatively by reducing the value of the lives of us all—say, by making truth antithetical to selfish individual motivation. What seems to be the most important is to have an adversary, not a colleague. Some adversaries are extreme and often the product of bigotry and/or psychosis, not always distinguishable one from the other.

Society as a whole, itself struggling inwardly, comes around to structuring itself along the lines of the "good" setting itself against the "bad." But ultimately even the best-organized social group crumbles when, as almost always happens, one or more group members turn against other group members under the weight of the predictable divisiveness that sets some members of a cohort against others, turning what could be friend into foe, Left against Right, white against black, old against young—identified and classified as to who is wrong and who is right, who owes the world what and what the world owes them, who has the power, who is the most moral, and who will drive whom out and away from the herd, never to be loved, to be left alone and not included. (An example of this process in action might be groups formed for the specific purpose of killing off opposing groups organized around such hot-button issues as abortion, liberalism, conservatism, and the like.)

A man in the majority of a particular society tells a man of a different race and religion "This is my town; time for you to get out" and does so in no uncertain terms, threatening to start a riot if there is lack of compliance. The first man thinks of himself as rational; pure adversarial cruelty is more to the point.

Leadership Issues

Fenichel says that Freud combined the speculative and the clinical bases "into a new instinct theory . . . which states that there are two qualities in the mind: a self-destructive one, the 'death instinct' (which can be turned toward the outside world and thus become a 'destructive instinct'), and an object-seeking quality, striving for higher units, the eros. The objection that in reality there is neither a pure self-destructive nor a pure object-seeking behavior is overcome by assuming that the real mental phenomena are composed of various 'mixtures' of these qualities."[14]

While some personality disorders seriously affect functionality, the admixture of Thanatos (the death instinct or desire to die) and Eros (the life instinct or desire to live) that is at times a feature of sadomasochism does not necessarily routinely reflect directly on an individual's personal and/or social functionality. What is important is to always keep in mind that sadomasochistically oriented individuals often have self-destructive and socially aggressive and loving elements mixed within their personality, and they can still function very well in certain arenas, that is, as highly competent autonomous adults, even as effective leaders, even though they internally object to what we would consider to be a positive outcome and externally do not entirely wish other individuals well. Such individuals can in certain situations, such as in politics (where being sadomasochistic—e.g., Machiavellian—can actually be contributory in a positive way), notably add to functionality and may even to a great extent be responsible for an individual's success and the high level of functionality of the group/society that he or she guides. In such cases curing sadomasochism may have a personal or even socially detrimental consequences. Generally, being self-defeating is not equal to the complexion of the whole patient; that is, the tendency to self-defeat doesn't characterize everything about a single patient, for sadomasochistic tendencies are often spotty. Patients who self-defeat and hurt others simultaneously often do so in certain segments of their lives only, leaving other sectors untouched and their overall functionality intact.

Still, this may be because the important positive advantages of sadomasochism even in its personally and socially self-destructive venues have not always been fully revealed to us even after probing hard, meant to divulge all its secrets. What is going on in this mysterious realm often remains an enigma and elusive even to the most astute student, who finds it very difficult to truly comprehend why someone, anyone, would act in a way that is antithetical to his or her own and others' ultimate best self-interests and what the benefits of acting this way are. This value of sadomasochism (like psychopathy) in a leader is a question that psychiatrists have struggled with for years and so far haven't convinced us or themselves that they know the answers. As Blum says, writing in his essay on masochism and trauma, "aspects of masochism continue to be mysterious, awaiting further illumination from multi-disciplinary research."[15] And one of these is the role sadomasochism can play in advancing causes as well as defeating goals. Some followers like having sadomasochists be their leader so that the leader who talks of giving his rivals body-slams has some on his side, while others are simply appalled by such brutality.

TREATMENT

Worse, we can't tell sadomasochists to simply stop it, the reason being that their own pressure to act one way or the other is not conscious but rather part of a personality disorder, and any personality disorder has unconscious roots, and that by definition is not something that is always and entirely subject to conscious control on anyone's part. How many times have I heard about a politician "If only he or she could stick to his agenda and stop the personal invective?" Yes, if only. But one can't stop a sadomasochistic personality (individual or group) disorder in its tracks just by wishing to do so any more than one can just stop one's OCPD or paranoia on command. Sadomasochists need to mistreat self and others in a way that amounts to torture to the point of one group attempting to destroy another not because they are making a conscious effort/choice to do so but because the id has taken over (fused with) the superego, self-destructing all concerned, if not on an individual level, then on a group level. Why would others who are friends compulsively need to mistreat other friends even of the same persuasion as their enemies as they suddenly give up on a person or a whole cadre of people they have known for years over something that is for every one of them of trivial personal or political significance? For the same reason perhaps that we hate another's successes and think we benefit the most from their failures: if there is no benefit there is at least some passing enjoyment in seeing our enemies squirm and go down, as Mark Altschule, a famous cardiologist, once said, "in a squashy heap." Why do we feel, or better, convince ourselves, that the world is a zero-sum place where one group to succeed must cause another group to fail and leave all concerned with zero status and zero physical (money in the bank) and personal (self-esteem) attributes in the psyche? Sadomasochism is close to schadenfreude.

We know that as for therapy of the individual, many sadomasochists do better with a noncritical therapist, one who avoids putting the patient down by emphasizing the more positive elements of the sadomasochistic patient's thoughts and actions—for example, you are not a bad person; you are just too anxious and afraid seemingly for your own good to be just too nice in many or all of your relationships.

Unlike those many other forms of therapy that are intentionally meant to be self-enhancing, therapy for sadomasochists should, at least sometimes/partially, be focused on *discouraging* the free expression of aspects of the true self. This is because for the sadomasochistic patient, self-realization often works against self-improvement. Indeed, the reverse pertains for the many sadomasochists who do best with therapists who tell them to keep their negativity inside and display only their less unseemly and more socially acceptable sides—for example, they as much as possible consider reducing displays of anger and resentment that distract from their basic nobility.

Too many sadomasochists, having become overly eager to sacrifice togetherness on the altar of the satisfaction of immediate negative emotional discharge, willingly relinquish being loved just in order to be triumphant—by allowing themselves to accept and validate all the knee-jerk responses that others hide. They gratify their need to hold back their anger, or express their anger sneakily, by refusing to alter spontaneously responses out of appropriate concern for what might happen next. As a result, for this more than almost any other kind of patient, self-mastery (not self-expression), often involving the conscious installation of self-control, becomes for them the royal road to self-improvement, especially in the important realm of the enhancement of their relationships with others.

Many sadomasochists respond to approaches that emphasize guilt reduction, while others (psychopathic/hypomanic sadomasochists) may benefit the most from approaches that emphasize the institution of self-control. Some sadomasochists respond effectively to insight therapy, but others, perhaps those less intellectually oriented, respond better to behavioral (action-oriented) approaches (e.g., approaches involving anger management).

All approaches that emphasize understanding and improving interpersonal relationships with the goal of helping one feel less lost, alone, and afraid are potentially helpful.

As a caveat, Reich says that "a definite dissolution of the masochistic character cannot take place until the patient has led an economic work and love life for a considerable period of time, that is, until long after the conclusion of the treatment."[16]

BIOLOGICAL (INHERENT) ASPECTS

Overall, it seems from a review of the literature that few observers have fully captured the essence of sadomasochism in the sense of not only the cause but also the ur-nature of self-defeat, individual or group, and so most people are unclear as to what to do to improve the individual and his or her world. Is sadomasochism in our genes? Is it the food chain operating? Is it as if the human organism has self-destruction as its fate, either because we desire our own death (as we have a death wish inside always working against us), wearing us out spontaneously, or even because we want to go along with it so that death is a process set off by the spark of life? Is there something self-destructive in the molecular structure of our protoplasm perhaps to be observed in/related to our psychology such as the too easy capacity for rage, as if rage is an in-built spontaneous (protective) device somewhat related to self-preservation? Or does it derive from our personal upbringing where parents' destructiveness takes the children down with them via a process of forced identification, the parents teaching the children to be unkind to self and others, to bully others as they bully each other, so that children grow up having been bullied in a way that gets passed down from generation to generation? Is it a personal hypersensitivity, a ur-neurosis that defeats us all? Or is it an acquired neurosis, just another Freudian tripartite construction, one standing comfortably beside obsessive-compulsive disorder or hysteria and therefore to be understood by studying self-destructiveness psychoanalytically, that is, from the dimensions of the interactions between the superego, ego ideal, ego, and id or, according to the dimensional viewpoint, following the pattern of any other personality disorder that is constructed out of bricks put together with the mortar of psychoanalytic concerns plus cognitive and interpersonal preoccupations? For some masochism is to be understood from the biological dimension, as a product of exhaustion as we give up the fight after struggling for just too many years with just too little to show for it to allow us to be ready to emerge robed for just one more battle against submission to what we are told is the inevitable attack by groups of the hostile persons all around us. Do we accept what we are told because we already feel this way ourselves?

2

Unique Characteristics of Sadomasochism

In its clinical manifestations, developmental patterns, and psychodynamic, experiential, social, and environmental qualities, self-defeating personality disorder/sadomasochism is characterized by unique imponderables, contradictions, and paradoxes that make it different from other psychoneuroses/psychoses. But though by nature this particular subject gives sadomasochism a unique quality that makes it different from other forms of mental illness, including other character disorders, it nevertheless retains its overlap with many of the other personality disorders, especially those marred by the agonies of depression and the suspiciousness of paranoia.

One unique aspect of self-defeating or sadomasochistic personality disorder is that patients actively seek failure in the face of every opportunity they might have to succeed. Another is that they actively seek to defeat the other individuals in their lives for reasons ranging from an innate generalized hostility to mankind to a specific desire to retaliate for feeling abandoned or controlled or being faced down by a competition that they believe is going to destroy them. In some ways, their behavior is not much different from the way all others with a neurosis behave toward themselves and others. In other ways, we recognize sadomasochism as a phenomenon different from other neurotic processes where the goal is to reduce pain and suffering and to come out whole. This difference perhaps accounts in great measure for the *DSM-5*'s failure to include sadomasochistic personality disorder in its compendium of personality disorders—those where the main goal seems to be not an intensification of hurtfulness all around but instead reduction of anxiety specifically attached to unique conflicts within oneself. Although this difference, covering such neurotic processes as obsessive-compulsive disorder (OCD) and hysteria, helps explain sadomasochism's general absence from the *DSM-5* compendium of personality disorders,[1] many of which run to type, in my opinion this is a difference without a distinction, representing as it does a true and serious absence of recognition and understanding. This seriously ultimately affects our ability to apply basic treatment methods valid for helping patients of today overcome a serious problem of living with others to enjoy the lives they have or could have had if only they would relinquish their need to suffer and remove a stop sign and instead put up one that says "Joy Ahead."

Another unique characteristic of sadomasochism is that where there is one psychodynamic there is also its opposite, often present in quality and quantity, accounting for much in the way of ambivalence and making sadomasochism a Janus-like disorder (i.e., one with two faces in its presentation). Thus, while there is a role played by social liberalism in sadomasochism (along the lines of anything goes), there is simultaneously one played by social conservatism in the presentation of the disorder (certain things are bad for you and for these you should be punished). Hence, some observers believe that sadomasochistic psychopathology thrives in a lax environment, while others see it as ingrained in the philosophy of a strict society (as a protest against excessive freedom). The sadomasochistic individual is paradoxically kind and cruel at one and the same time. Thus, the sadomasochistic OCD who dirties the house to annoy his mate is in some ways simultaneously constantly straightening out things with the same purpose in mind (including self-torture and torturing his or her buddy).

Another involves the predominance of the chicken-or-egg which comes first type of controversy when referring to the clinical picture. Thus, one book, Chancer's *Sadomasochism in Everyday Life*,[2] puts forth a hypothesis that she feels is highly relevant to a discussion of mental illness in general and the personality disorders in particular: the idea that primary individual sadomasochism—and the self-defeating personality whose path it traces—is (analyzable along Freudian lines and Reich's concepts of character armoring) what generates our sadomasochistic social culture, characterized by groupings and marked by everyday experiences of aggressive dominance alternating with abject subordination to others of like mind.

But (and as with all that is sadomasochistic) an opposite theory also exists: the possibility that it is our social culture that generates individual sadomasochism. Thus, Chancer notes Fromm's "sense of sadomasochism as a strategy adopted to defend ourselves from socially rooted anxieties."[3] Do video games create/catalyze sadomasochistic behavior, or does personal endogenous sadomasochistic behavior catalyze the content of video games?

Also unique is the extent to which sadomasochism and normalcy are on a continuum. Sadomasochism on the one hand bears a close clinical relationship to normal behavior, so that one never knows where exactly to draw the line between normative anger and abnormal hatred, the ordinary and the exceptional rages we all have. Sadomasochism also has a special relationship to everyday social phenomena, which means that everywhere we turn we see the cruelty of self-defeat and of defeating others in action, with all concerned relatively helpless to protect themselves from the onslaught of those who would wish us ill, those often but not always the same people who act upon their negativity and turn others' lives, and ultimately their own, into exercises of misery and deprivation imposed from within and without. Recently, I have heard over and over again that certain people are so nasty these days that others leave them, crying and hoping to never see them ever again. Political arguments in particular sometimes represent not discussions but pitched battles, and the hope that we can have civilized debate fades with each day of some political campaigns. The conclusion is inevitable: sadomasochism is so much a variant of normal that it is found at least to some degree in almost everybody at all times. We all get depressed from time to time, and we all blame the other person for our own misfirings much as all of us with paranoid tendencies project our own dysfunctions onto others, leaving us with the view that we are purportedly free of any self-created emotional problems. And cruelty to others is present, hopefully in latent form, in the inner workings of all of us. The distance between narcissism and altruism is like the distance between the two poles of a horseshoe: one travels a long distance along the path from one end to another only to wind up essentially at the same place we started. One can indeed see Russia from Alaska.

Secrecy is a hallmark of this disorder. When it comes to clinical evaluation, sadomasochists, like many other patients with an emotional disorder, are a maddeningly uncooperative group with a seriously disruptive tendency to be as untruthful with their therapists as they are with everyone else, including themselves. According to the experts, speaking of psychopaths in words easily adaptable to the evaluation of sadomasochists, they are even able to fake the results of psychological tests such as the MMPI and the Rorschach without too much difficulty in order to impress, cow, or manipulate the tester. Liking themselves the way they are, they do so to make certain that all concerned find it frustrating because they are unable/unwilling to tell us what we need to know to understand them and help them change. Thus, they can't or won't answer such questions as "Why would anybody be loath to strive to be successful but instead try to achieve the opposite: ignominy, shame, dishonor, and disgrace?" While many neurotics are eager to speak up about themselves with the goal of self-improvement, many sadomasochists are eager to cover up how they work internally because they don't understand what they are dealing with or, understanding it, are loath to reveal how they operate, if only because they are too ashamed of themselves to reveal the powers that afflict them and make them who and what they are, both morally and sexually, thus turning them into the monsters that some of them act like or can in fact be.

The possible biological nature of sadomasochism is unique to this disorder. That is, it is possible that sadomasochistic tendencies are in our DNA, raising the possibility that this is an issue not of neurosis but instead of temperament, which is inborn. Perhaps this means that no psychological study of this issue will bring up very much, accounting for our general inability to sink our teeth into this behavior to get a real feel for what is going on in its ephemeral far reaches. Maybe sadomasochism is best conceptualized as one of the components of, one of the links in, the biological food chain and thus is not a purely psychological issue involving the psyche (i.e., the superego; the ego instincts, such as hunger; the ego ideal, such as what I want or demand out of my life; and the id, such as the base, pure instincts of sex and aggression) but instead is nature's way of digging and paving the road to survival, and not necessarily of the fittest, thus getting something to eat. Can anyone really understand why the dog and the cat don't always get along? Can anyone really understand why snake charmers are born, not made?

There is also a willfulness (ego-syntonicity) about sadomasochism that differentiates it from a disease that is impossible to tame or a disorder that begs to be cured. Fewer people seem to say about OCD "this is me" than do people who identify with their sadomasochistic personality traits and accept them as being "who I am" so that sadomasochists don't buy into the suggestion that they would be almost anything else if they only could be, making sadomasochism an ego-syntonic (e.g., wanted) disorder. The question then arises, is sadomasochistic behavior willful, or can sadomasochists help themselves no more than the patient who is hungry or a diabetic can take his or her eyes off the chocolate-covered cookie in the bins at the supermarket?

There is a controversy as to whether the motivation for sadomasochists in treatment is to bare their soul and thereby get better through insight or to keep their little peccadilloes—say, about their self-defeating tendencies—and stay the same. In this respect too unlike most neurotic disorders, often sadomasochistic seems more like a preference than a problem. The continuum between normal and pathological sadomasochism is thus even smoother and tighter than we sometimes perceive it to be.

Fewer legal implications pertain with most other neurotic disorders. Here, however, certain behaviors can get the involved individual into real trouble, making sadomasochism seem in some cases more like a criminal activity (badness) than like an emotional compulsion/illness.

Family and friends are often extensively involved in the fallout of the disorder, for unlike such neuroses as OCD this is not primarily a private matter. Like passive-aggression, it takes at least two to nurture sadomasochism, making it primarily a dyadic disorder. Sadomasochists can and do rule harshly over the family as a whole and have especially negative effects because there is a significant component of shame associated with the disorder, so that one person focuses all his or her wrath not merely on him or herself but also on one or more chosen targets who bear the brunt in a close, almost airtight relationship between two people along the lines of "Who exactly is hurting whom, who started it, and who plans to go on doing so? I'll never tell."

Widespread identifiable social involvements do exist and of necessity are sometimes more than prevailingly modest, and there is a tendency to use rationalization to explain them. Thus, the sadomasochist will say about his or her spouse, "He/she deserves it; he/she brought it upon him/herself," but the socially active sadomasochist almost always says, "I am doing this for the benefit of the world, no matter how much it negatively affects me personally. I am not a person with social problems; I am the One sent here to solve them. Sometimes I am the conservative here to control the liberal; sometimes I am the liberal here to rein in the conservative."

Comparatively, the only other disorder with such social implications as self-defeating personality disorder is psychopathy. Relatively speaking, while most other psychiatric diagnoses focus on individual behavior with only secondary concern for the social impact of that behavior, a diagnosis of sadomasochistic personality disorder or self-defeating personality disorder is more heavily imbued with and fundamentally rests and depends upon social interactions that become interwoven into the fabric of the disorder, sometimes to a significant extent. A central concept when discussing sadomasochistic personality disorder is therefore its social implications. As with psychopaths, one of the most important criteria of sadomasochistic personality disorder is its antisocial hostility toward others. But unlike psychopathy, sadomasochism is a uniquely socially approved behavior, as it is becoming more and more acceptable to act violent with someone with whom we disagree, thereby becoming personally one of our most vocal personality assets and politically its possession coming across not as self-defeating but instead as self-improving. Also, sadomasochism has become far more relevant to the here and now than is a disorder such as obsessive-compulsive personality disorder (OCPD) that takes us back to our early history (e.g., our early toilet training). Though it can be done, we are hard-pressed to firmly relate the former to anything in the child's early life and experiences with his parents when he was a child.

Is sadomasochism a defense neurosis, that is, related to the reduction of anxiety, or is it something else? Fromm and Reich would disagree.

Chancer, referring to Fromm, notes that that while other disorders may or may not resemble childishness in some key ways, the applicability of the comparison between sadomasochism and the Freudian tripartite model of neurosis is weak: the overlap between childishness (regression) is less striking and significant than is the resemblance between, say, histrionic behavior and being childish, being paranoid and being childish, and so on insofar as sexuality and other relational matters are concerned.

Observers such as Fromm believe that anxiety is not a predominant feature of sadomasochism, so Freud's tripartite model hardly applies. Thus, according to Chancer, Fromm believes that sadomasochism is a strategy adopted to defend ourselves from socially rooted anxieties. Also according to some observers, sadomasochism appears as a fundament, rooted in biology as a primary pursuit of actual pleasure more so than as an avoidance of neurotic pain. The goal of getting what you want involves less a reduction of anxiety than an acquisition of something alluring, something good to have for yourself. For sadomasochism, the expression "revenge is sweet" is far more applicable than it might be for a disorder such as OCPD, where revenge is a modest, if nonexistent, element in the process.

Thus, according to theorists such as Fromm, sadomasochism is not so much tied in with the manifestations of the defense mechanisms as are other psychological disorders. With OCD there is doing and undoing as the defense mechanism fundamental to the process, and with hysteria there is repression. But with sadomasochism one is dealing more with an unhealthy breakthrough of fundamental primitive energy (such as that bound up in temperament) than with suppression of a disavowed frightening wish at the behest of anxiety so that sadomasochism is more like a simple process of discharge than a complex resolution of conflict. Many view this disorder as one emphasizing various manifestations of fundamental (primary) guilt rather than as one of the employment of mechanisms to deal with anxiety. In this regard, many view it not as an anxiety-driven conflict originating in the id versus the superego but instead as a primary urge, much like primary narcissism, or the essentially unexplainable emotions of love and hate, and so very much unlike other neurotic or psychotic disorders that are clinical manifestations of active conflict. In short, for these authors sadomasochism is something that is natively endowed, more as part of one's nature than part of the scenario of one's nurture.

While Fromm sees sadomasochistic individuals not as natively "endowed," as such possessed of a life-force that is primary, and as having developed "a strategy adopted to defend [themselves] from socially rooted anxieties," Reich applies the Freudian model with a twist of his own. For Reich, the resultant product of emotional stress is not called a "neurotic symptom" but instead is what he calls the "character armor."[4] Attempts to relate sadomasochism developmentally to orality, anality, and the phallic eras of child development continue to be made (e.g., particularly by Cooper[5] and Kernberg[6] in their writings), but they can seem incomplete unless accompanied by satisfying alterative explanations, particularly those of the psychology of the here and now. Still, while many observers connect sadomasochism in adulthood with sadomasochism in childhood (e.g., with the parental behavior, or input from the parents), such connections are not so overt as the presumed relationship between other psychoneuroses and issues related to childhood development. Early dependency, toilet training, and oedipal conflicts assume less center stage here than in the developmental protocol for a neurosis such as OCD.

The element of controversy as to the origins of sadomasochism is astounding. Some observers say of sadomasochism that in their background sadomasochists were as children overgratified, so some are still looking for that stroking they once had, while others say sadomasochists as children were undergratified and are highly invested now in making up for what they never had or for the love they have subsequently now lost. Most observers before making the diagnosis of a personality disorder require that the personality-disordered behaviors in question started in adolescence or earlier. No such constraints appear to be required for making the diagnosis of sadomasochistic personality disorder. Sadomasochism, like post-traumatic stress disorder (PTSD), is not necessarily a problem appearing earlier in life such as might be with avoidant personality disorder. This characterological disorder is not so clearly evident by early childhood or so invariably chronic throughout life. Very often sadomasochism may involve a transitional change, not an enduring personality change, even one that can result from catastrophic events, constituting a kind of reactive disorder that appears in the adult after trauma and is akin to, or one subtype of, PTSD (such as put forth in the theory of life psychology).

MORAL MASOCHISM

Sadomasochism is not necessarily a sexual issue. Also, it is not as much a moral problem as is psychopathy. The psychopath might say, "If it brings me benefit [if it feels good], do it," though it is immoral, while the sadomasochist might say, "My giving myself a go-ahead to obtain pleasure has nothing to do with morality, good or bad."

But sadomasochism does elicit more moral judgment than the hand washing of OCPD or the paralyzed arm of hysteria. The comparison between sadomasochists/sadomasochism and evil and the expressed belief that sadomasochists are evil people is generally more prominently made/sustained more than ordinarily so when it comes to the study of other mental illnesses.

Sadomasochism rarely gets into the stream of using a disorder as an insanity defense, as might, for example, schizophrenia or bipolar disorder. Many people prefer to view the sadomasochist as bad rather than as sick. This is especially true of sexual sadomasochism and derives in particular from one's attitude that sex itself is bad, even when performed in the missionary position within marriage. Sexual sadomasochism is almost always seen as immoral and is usually believed to be a victimless crime.

For severe cases, treatment controversies exist as well, particularly whether treatment should take place in an open or closed facility where therapists can have all features of the patient under observation and whether one should consider a permissive or constrained atmosphere for the patient. Most other disorders, psychopathy and borderline conditions in particular, are at some point in their development considered for inpatient treatment. Sadomasochism is rarely on this list.

3

More Unique Characteristics of Sadomasochism

The *DSM-5* presents a confused picture of sadomasochism as either being or not being a true personality disorder. The *DSM-5* does not view sadomasochism as constituting a true personality disorder compared to other personality disorders in that its chief characteristic involves thoughts and actions that are strikingly both self-defeating *and* generally simultaneously hurtful to others. Though such a compound formation is striking and though we all experience sadomasochistic movement within ourselves, officially, however, sadomasochism, as previously noted, is not in the *DSM-5* as one of the personality disorders. Sadomasochism is not considered to be a valid, recognizable, reliably identifiable conglomerate of traits able to be precisely spotted by diverse clinicians, each independently and accurately pinpointing its unique qualities while ignoring supposed artifacts that contaminate the picture and confuse the definitive "official" models and concepts. A specific identifiable syndrome, one that is essentially different from all the others, is not believed to exist for those who manifest characteristic sadomasochistic traits. For others, with careful observation and moving the goalpost just a little bit, a definitive process does emerge with clear, characteristic features.

Though sadomasochistic personality disorder is not even referenced in the index of the *DSM-5*, the *DSM-5* does supply two categories for two situations where it could potentially fit in:

- The individual's personality pattern meets the general criteria for a personality disorder, and traits of several different personality disorders are present, but the criteria for any specific personality disorder are not met.
- The individual's personality pattern meets the general criteria for a personality disorder, but the individual is considered to have a personality disorder that is not included in the *DSM-5* classification (e.g., sadomasochistic personality disorder).

The *DSM-5* does describe sadomasochistic *tendencies* under the heading "paraphiliac disorders," which include sexual masochism disorder (humiliation, bondage, or suffering) and sexual sadism disorder (inflicting humiliation, bondage, or suffering on others).

Virtually no distinction is made in the *DSM-5* between the emotional and physical components of sadomasochistic fantasies/behavior. The two are seen as fusing (e.g., as "preferential"), though the concept of moral masochism (unaccompanied by sexual sadism), to continue to exist, would have to favor separating each, however much they overlap clinically.

This said, some authors, dynamically speaking, lay emphasis upon the presence or absence of guilt, returning sadomasochism to what we believe to be its rightful place among the personality disorders. The concept of sadomasochism representing a compromise formation and an anxiety reducer returns this disorder to what should be its familiar place in the legion of the anxiety neuroses along Freud's tripartite vision of a mental disorder being the product of id, creating guilt managed by invoking a neurotic symptom such as the paralyzed arm of the hysteric as a compromise between expressing and holding back anger.

Generally, psychosocial impairment is, if not entirely overlooked, not applied when it is indicated and proper to do so.

Not surprisingly the relationship between hurtful sadomasochistic fantasies and other related or unrelated sources of pathology (in the form of such comorbidity as obsessiveness) is underplayed. While the concept of comorbidity is present, it is here defined as representing the *concomitant* presence of other disorders (e.g., the affiliation of sadomasochism with alcohol and substance misuse disorders), but the blending of two or more disorders leading to a difficulty/inability to distinguish one disorder from the other within a mash made up of symptomatic or nonsymptomatic clinical overlap—for example, that between obsessive-compulsive personality disorder (OCPD), paranoia, and sadomasochism—is not discussed.[1]

Sadomasochism presents itself differently from case to case, as the manifest clinical behaviors, being a unique mash, differ from patient to patient. In all sadomasochists, as Reich says, offering us a general description of the problem, their sadomasochism is composed of traits that belong to other disorders, here selected specifically to combine to constitute this singular piece of pathology. That is, while according to Reich the main "traits of sadomasochism are found, individually, in all neurotic characters, [together] they form the sadomasochistic character only when they are all present, and when they determine the key to the personality and its typical reactions."[2]

Reich would specify how sadomasochism presents itself in different ways from case to case. What varies is the specific selection of sadomasochistic building blocks (components) as they differ from patient to patient dependent on the ones chosen from other disorders to form the final picture. Inconstant behaviors that present or are elicited include restricted gratifications (borrowed from depression, etc.); the specific manifestation of self-harm, such as self-cutting or not eating; head banging or breath holding; the preference for a specific paragenital sexual act; the degree of great shame that causes or accompanies these various behaviors; a general need to fail in life; specific self-defeating resistance and professional behaviors, such as always being late to work or marital and family battles; excessively feeling blue and pessimistic; too quiet a life to contain much enjoyment; a poor sense of humor; overconscientiousness; and being too reliable and extensively responsible for too much, combined with rigidly maintained negative self-judgment vis-à-vis even the slightest peccadillo, with typical negative self-devaluation here too if one doesn't live up to one's own and others' moral and practical standards and demands. Aspirations are denied; talents are neglected; people are allowed or encouraged to humiliate a victim (oneself or others); innocent questions in either direction are allowed to pass as attacks (the paranoid tendency to respond to innocent questions as if they are attacks); problematic life situations go unchallenged and unchanged, as when they are accepted as normal or inevitable; and pathological going along with frustrating destructive or demeaning work situations occurring with need for change are ignored due to conventional ideology's saying the equivalent of "tough it out," "it's bad to be happy on your job, for work is work," "some of the worst jobs are overall the best jobs out there either for financial reasons or for future potential advancement," and "work is not a reason for fun." A friend wanted her ashes scattered over the ocean and asked if I would do it; she then added, "Me and my dogs too." Someone asked, "Are you going to have your dogs killed so that they can join you in the death scatter too?" And she never spoke to that person again, presumably for his having accused her of being that kind of person who would think of her as someone doing such a dirty deed. How was that person to know that the dogs she meant were in an urn in the other room, having been cremated years ago and ready to be scattered when the time was right.

This said, the main component in the forefront of the clinical picture of sadomasochism continues to be the attainment of pleasure through the infliction of pain. This applies either to oneself or toward another individual, so that one might inflict pain on oneself and/or inflict pain on another or do both simultaneously or sequentially.

The mechanism whereby pain is inflicted is complicated in large measure because a half-full/half-empty duality exists between pleasure and pain. Thus, one can inflict pain actively by the direct induction of pain or passively by hurting another by ignoring that singular person, thereby depriving that person of pleasure, perhaps the same pleasure offered to another. One can "inflict" pleasure by the induction of pleasure directly (e.g., giving a degree of satisfaction/pleasure by giving him or her a massage) and/or by arranging for someone malleable to accept desired pain.

So, clinically, typical sadomasochistic character traits, are according to Reich, "subjectively, a chronic sensation of *suffering* which appears objectively as a *tendency to complain;* chronic tendencies to *self-damage* and *self-depreciation* ('moral sadomasochism') and a compulsion to *torture others* which makes the patient suffer no less than the object." Post-traumatic stress disorder is a well-known example of self-inflicted sadomasochism which has a primary or secondary effect on others.[3] Many sadomasochistic characters show a specifically awkward, atactic (uncoordinated) behavior in their manners and in their intercourse with others, often one so marked as to give the impression of mental deficiency.

Like any other character attitude, the sadomasochistic attitude shows not only in interpersonal relationships but also in the inner life of the person, which can, for example, be equally chaotic. Dynamically speaking, attitudes that originally were relevant to other people are maintained in the conscience toward these other people who as of now have been introjected. Thus, the next step: what was originally external and then became internalized must again be externalized in the (analytic) transference so that behavior that is first acquired in infancy shows in adulthood in the relationship with others, often one after the other. A mother who makes a child eat his or her hated broccoli or wear wool clothes when the child is allergic to lanolin can easily reappear in adulthood as the sadistic dietician, the clothier who favors garments that fit too tightly to allow one to breathe comfortably/properly, or the other clothier who dresses the child in wool suits that itch. The witch is an example of the regurgitated hostile mother who can do practically anything destructive and whose primary purpose is to do so to his or her children.

One way sadomasochistic personality possibilities/disorder can be differentiated from nonsadomasochistic personality problems/disorders is by the way patients with the different personality disorders each handles his or her anger. As with many sadomasochistic phenomena, moderation is not necessarily part of the picture. In the self-defeating patient suffering from the sadomasochism of everyday life, parents are often blamed for everything by a sadistic child (sadistic children) who goes astray, and the parents often illegitimately blame themselves for everything (e.g., "where did I go wrong?"). Conversely, parents often blame "bad children" for their own problem when in fact it is the parents who started it.

A woman has three children by two marriages. Her children refuse to see her because she doesn't admit what she has done wrong to them. Worse, according to them, she refuses to admit it in writing, which is the only way they will accept her apologies, if even then. She then sends out the following e-mail: "See me by June first for after that I will be dead." No one comes. On June 2 she commits suicide after shooting up a house of worship.

Sadomasochism is often conscious. As with other things psychological, the unconscious, using such defenses as reaction formation ("I am only hoping for the best for you"), clicks in to reduce tension, which is the product of anxiety and guilt. But sadomasochism may not strictly speaking be a defense mechanism; it is not as automatic as are the defense mechanisms associated with other neuroses. For example, a sadomasochist uses the defense mechanism of rationalization, which is not an automatic entry into sadomasochistic boundaries and as a sticky reminder within the sadomasochistic portal as is projection, so that when such individuals come to a certain psychological trigger/psychic crossroads they dredge up a readily available sadomasochism to automatically guide their way. As a result, sadomasochists are often at least semiaware of why they do what they do, and they don't see why they should stop it. A phallic sadomasochistic woman gives her neighbor a requested recipe; unconsciously, however, she fails to include one important ingredient of the recipe: the asparagus. She does what is expected of her mostly but not entirely and without full knowledge of what she is doing and how she is being harmful, unconsciously, to a beloved friend and his family. As an obsessional such a person might say "I forgot" (and actually truly mean it), but as a sadomasochist such a person may say "that'll teach her for trying to mooch in on my secrets."

All emotional illnesses have an unconscious sadomasochistic quality to them; conversely, when one detects sadomasochism on any level, one should get beyond the diagnosis of sadomasochism and make a differential diagnosis. Three distinctions that should especially be made are the ones between sadomasochism and paranoid personality disorder, narcissistic personality disorder, and borderline personality disorder.

Patients with a depressive personality component take their anger out on themselves and do so directly clinically in a way that is generally obvious to even the most remote and uninvolved of observers (e.g., depressives themselves don't see their anger and thus take it out on themselves). In contrast, patients with paranoid tendencies reattribute their anger so that instead of getting angry and becoming depressed, paranoid individuals take their anger out on others so as to scrub their own anger clean as not being part of themselves after redistributing their anger so that their anger takes form in a projective belief that "others are responsible for the bad things that are happening to me [projection] and make me angry." Finally, some sadomasochistic patients are pretty obviously angry people, angry about everything, but seeing clearly what they are angry about and why, have many compunctions about letting others know that's how they feel, and treating themselves and everyone else accordingly—hurtfully discharging their pain openly, either on themselves as masochism or on others as sadism, or as both, as sadomasochism. Fights ensue.

These individuals are as adept at tormenting others as they are at tormenting themselves with anger. Conversely, any symptoms wherein an individual consciously or unconsciously limits pleasure and unpleasure in an (unconsciously) motivated and automatic way can belong here, the obligatory limiting of pleasure and the infliction of pain to all being if not the commonest then at least the most serious of sadomasochistic manifestations.

Issues of self-esteem contribute to the picture of one individual's sadomasochism. Sadomasochists enhance their self-esteem while sacrificing others to their own needs, or they set about lowering the self-esteem of all concerned, others, and their own. Low self-esteem in sadomasochism is discussed throughout this book.

Many sadomasochists have a need to get attention through displayed disability. For others, often denial accompanies the defense of rationalization. These sadomasochists rarely think of themselves as ill (i.e., as deficient psychologically). In the latter case, ego-syntonicity of their sadomasochism is primary, which means they like themselves the way they are and so readily excuse everything they do.

Though various sadomasochists display different profiles, which may be ones of detachment, hurtfulness, disinhibition, and psychoticism, all include unconscious negative affectivity and antagonism somewhere in the clinical picture. Depressive sadomasochistic individuals are particularly antagonistic to, as much as they are detached from, others. And many are more inhibited than disinhibited in their anger.

Though derangement syndromes are common, sadomasochists rarely display symptoms of primary psychoticism. It would appear, however, that all psychoticism routinely has a sadomasochistic component to it.

In social psychoticism (which is generally a derangement syndrome), a defined society welcomes and reflects individual/group sadomasochism (as happens with some cults in a pseudopsychotic fashion). For these individuals the psychotic components of sadomasochism (often those of a sexual nature) are particularly appealing or useful, though others prefer bland while others prefer horrifying interactions. (The séance as once practiced with a bloody white cock exemplifies this.) A feature of sadomasochistic derangement is delusional thinking whereby a patient creates adversarial relationships out of little to nothing so that the lyrics to the song "Baby It's Cold Outside" are read as referring to male dominance of women—an implication of Berne's "rapo"[4] involving not letting a date go home in a timely fashion but in effect chaining her to the bedpost or binding her with twine or masking tape and raping her in a bloody fashion (in no sense being welcoming for this person as something desirable).

This said, sometimes sadomasochistic derangement brings out the best in other people. At a coffeehouse I frequent a schizophrenic man passes much of his time hanging out dining on the free coffee and food treats the management gives him, loudly talking to himself and laughing at the air. He must certainly take away some of the establishment's business as the customers leave because of his behavior, but management gives him free food and drink out of the goodness of their hearts in what I consider to be one of the blessed features of being masochistic and, some would say, to a masochistic derangement (self-sacrificial) degree. (The manager thinks she can handle him by simply telling him to "zip up your mouth" when he becomes too rambunctious, but this only works intermittently and mostly causes him to escalate.) Also, in the backstory of derangement syndromes is that some societies welcome and reflect individual derangement for its more appealing components (e.g., the good witch or the merry tutelary), so they say nothing bad about some of the more "evil" features of such rituals as Halloween celebrations.

Clearly, in trying to spot sadomasochism we should not overlook the purely descriptive/behavioral approach to determining this diagnosis, one based almost entirely on observed, manifest (clinical) features. Too limited an approach would involve focusing on the central defining, *dynamic* issues that characterize this disorder. What Stricker[5] says is an exception here: the diagnosis of sadomasochistic personality disorder should be made not only on the basis of the manifest behavior but also on the basis of the dynamisms of that behavior, for dynamic issues tend to be more fundamental and lead to greater pathognomonic differentiation than do purely descriptive presentations/evaluations. If we equate stubbornness with anality, we might diagnose OCPD when the true diagnosis is sadomasochistic personality disorder simply because we have a reductionistic mind-set that tells us to look for anxiety over guilty wishes when in any given cases our mind-set here may be primarily the wish to be hurtful, vengeful, spiteful, and retaliatory: at last we have found our opportunity to get back at someone for a hurt he or she inflicted on us some years ago. Therapeutic interventions follow. With sadomasochists it is true that the elephant that stomps its trainer may not be the elephant who is fearful but rather the elephant who remembers.

4

The Sadomasochism of Everyday Life

Negative and Positive Aspects

NEGATIVE VALUES

The role that anger plays in the sadomasochism of everyday life is chiefly determined by the role it plays in the formation and maintenance of sadomasochism in all venues. We cannot meaningfully discuss individual sadomasochism in isolation from its overall negative and positive manifestations in both interpersonal and social arenas, including its domestic and socioeconomic manifestations and implications, ranging from marital sadomasochism to the sadomasochism inherent in the political sphere (as reflected, for example, in the sadomasochism sometimes coming out of the White House and written about, often excessively and exclusively, in the daily news).

I believe that anger is in all of us and that we all get into the anger loops characteristic of sadomasochism that go round and round until the bubble bursts and there is discharge in one form (symptom) or another. The actual manifestations of the discharge depend on the nature of the provocation of the anger, the self-control potential/manifest, and the response of others to the seething or outbursts such as there may be. Angry moral motivations may prevail, or the anger may from the start have a sexual implication as a kiss turns into a bite or deteriorates in fantasy or, in reality, into something more intensive. In those cases where accusations of past sexual harassment exist, the spirit of the complaints may be accurate; in other cases they are not what they seem to be because they arise out of personal animus—malevolent sadomasochistic fantasies as much as any reality that ever existed. In some cases of accusations of past sexual harassment, fantasies arise to meet expectations, being somewhat distortive-symbolic. The masochist expects to be mistreated and instead of calling closeness "attention" or "love" calls it "harassment." False memories often of a paranoid nature can develop and take the form of critical attacks on innocent parties. In metanoia, which is reverse paranoid sadomasochism, the repression of actual attacks can spare guilty parties the comeuppance they deserve.

An interesting concept is that of a syndrome related to being sophomoric, the Hubris Syndrome. Owen and Davidson describe this disorder as "the ability to make swift decisions, sometimes based on little evidence." If a leader and thin-skinned, the person with this syndrome "will not be able to stand the process of public scrutiny, attacks by opponents, and back-stabbings from within, without some form of self-exultation and grand belief about their own mission and importance."[1]

Here are some examples of sadomasochism in everyday life that are universal, contain elements of this syndrome, and are therefore likely to be troublesome enough to require paying attention to one's own psychological distortions followed by outside intervention directed toward countering this syndrome and, in the political world at the very least, thinking twice about voting for someone suffering from this disordered mind-set.

Sadomasochism at Home

Sadomasochistic mothers. The following letter, sent on a very important holiday to others who were presumably having a good time, illustrates the multiple levels of sadomasochism in everyday life. Here we have a mother using a holiday-crafted letter to beat a friend over her head with the mother's own bloody body, a letter that also illustrates the relationship between sadism (to the recipient of the letter) and masochism (using one's ruminative "poor little me" suffering in order to inflict pain or further pain upon oneself).

This self-sacrificial mother writes:

> I am kind of shell-shocked by the way my three children turned out. Jane and I are civil and pleasant to each other, but will only be peripheral to each other's lives. Peter never comes over or calls and just recently I discovered

> he got married without even telling me. Sandy in no way repays all the sacrifices I made for him by my volunteering at the schools so that he would be treated well by the teachers, and paying for lessons in wood-working, dancing, arts and crafts, gymnastics, karate, tennis, swimming, as well as the basketball camps we sent him to. And what about the baseball and softball we played together and the times we spent building snow dinosaurs; cooking together; going to play groups; my driving him to golf-coaching lessons; taking him to plays in children's and adult theater, having extended family dinners every Sunday so that he would get a sense of belonging and feeling important; giving him cello lessons and guitar lessons and everything else he wanted to do so that he would be able to find out what he loved and determine his own identity. Hey, Sandy, all the trips we took you on—to England because you loved the Beatles, to Hawaii, France, Italy, and Disney World because you loved all their songs?
>
> But you, and all of you kids, decided you hated us, your parents, anyway. On second thought, you are NOT welcome back, you sorry excuses for kids. Shame on all of you and I am sick of bearing the consequences of your lack of character and appreciation. All I can say is I think I was a complete failure as a parent. (Why not, 'You are a complete failure as a child'?)

Sadomasochistic children. More and more instances of children abandoning their parents seem to be coming to our attention in recent years and have hurtful implications in the extreme. The example that infuriates some of us the most is that of the adopted child who has been brought up lovingly and expensively by his or her new parents, who saved his or her life, only to come out of it with "what I want out of life is to find my real mother"—talk about ingratitude. The usual response on the parents' part is to beg, accompanied by protestations that I always loved you as much as your biological mother ever would have done, followed by questions such as "why are you doing this to me?" This naturally only intensifies the child's participation in this sadomasochistic game. I have found that if the parents simply refuse to participate in this ongoing sadomasochistic enmeshment, things improve, and if they stop wringing their hands, things improve, and they do so sometimes very rapidly; the first sign is a phone call from the child along the lines of "Is everything all right? I am worried about you." Of course, what some of these children are worried about is whether or not they have done their parent some real damage that they ultimately can't live with. Fighting this sadism with masochism rarely works; a proper response may be to maintain one's distance until the child's panic level of regret becomes intolerable. Timing is, however, of great importance: too soon and the approach hasn't had enough time to work; too late and the kids are probably already in therapy working on "parents as enemies." But it is unlikely that in therapy they are trying to find out what they can do to be better children vis-à-vis their deserving (adoptive) parents; it is more likely that they are coming forth with an orgy of complaints about how their parents mistreated them and what they can do to avoid them and still be named in the will. Cases of blame-the-victim are in the making.

Sadomasochistic fathers. A father hired his son to work for him and then acted out a sadomasochistic oedipally tinged father-son rivalry because he, the father, wanted to be top dog, regardless of how this affected his son and what it did to the business. The father deliberately weakened the son by assigning him to do the things the son hated to do. Once he even put the son in "Siberia," an out-of-the-way warehouse where he sent him to supervise all the other intractable workers, most of whom were themselves already there because they had done something the boss felt warranted their banishment. Basically, this was the father's way to get revenge on his son for his being younger and stronger than he, the father, was. The father's brother went along as a way to gain further advantage over and to get revenge on the victim for being the rival sibling whose rivalry had successful components. As a masochist, the son went along, giving in and self-damaging in order to avoid doing some personal and professional damage to the company, which also paid his salary. The entire eye-for-an-eye plan backfired; soon enough all three stopped seeing each other socially and then stopped speaking to each other professionally as well (at work). No business got done, and a year afterward the business folded completely.

A healthy approach would have been to improve oneself and one's work until the situation balanced out, with the son's value to the business recognized as too impressive to be sacrificed on the pyre of some petty intellectual oedipally tinged battleground.

Sadomasochistic marriages (and divorce). Everyday life is filled with subtle sadomasochistic provocations within relationships. A sadomasochistic personality disorder should only be diagnosed if such behavior becomes habitual. Ongoing sadomasochistic provocations are, I believe, the chief reason for a divorce. In fact, divorce itself is a sadomasochistic interaction and outcome between two people. Rarely are the *issues* thoroughly discussed before a divorce; emotions always get into it, and ongoing anger is generally the chief driving passion on a recurrent basis. I believe that the best way to prevent a divorce is to see it as the accumulation of literally hundreds of sadomasochistic daily mininegative interactions. Each member of the marital dyad should be aware of this pattern and alert to how easily created good relationships routinely get contaminated by bad sadomasochistic atrocities, however minor. When not of major proportions, these aggravations may consist of trivial oral deprivations (of dependency needs), simple control issues (telling a perfectly mature adult the one right thing to do when things can be done another way just as efficiently and profitably, there being more than one valid approach to doing some things), and close-to-original oedipal struggles so that triangular situations develop where there is jealousy (often deliberately provoked because "if you are jealous of me that means that you love me"). These line up, reinforce each other, and accumulate until a straw breaks the camel's back, and in a version of Berne's game of Uproar[2] (one of his many essentially sadomasochistic games), the situation explodes, and there is no going back, especially when things are said and done to deliberately elicit fear and anger on a victim's part and sincere regrets are later left unexpressed. This is the remedy: decide that you don't want a divorce first, then sift all interactions through the filter of unsadomasochism, which allows for the repair of sadomasochistic dyadic contacts/squelches and provocations immediately as they occur so there is no accumulation of resentment. The overall goal is to never hurt another person, and that person includes first your significant other and then yourself.

You already know what annoys a partner; stop doing it and in a virtuous cycle the relationship likely improves and divorce is avoided. My principle is this: your first marriage should be your last marriage if possible, because most of the time serial marriages do not involve progressive improvement, and the next is rarely a bettering of the first object choice you make, because though the first time you are still young and inexperienced, most people ultimately don't differ that much, so even thinking of looking for someone else better involves attempting to improve on something that is likely to be in the first place just as good as it will ever get. So, turn the relationship you have around by eliminating repetitive sadomasochistic provocations until you see your relationship in a totally different light, and you will likely no longer have that much of a reason to abandon what you already have. Especially watch out for the hidden small provocations. Just recently I was at a wedding party where the hostess got up, said she had an appointment to help a girlfriend exercise, and left the proceedings without so much as saying a good-bye to the bride or the groom. Why did she make this arrangement in the first place? Will the couple ever forget the impression of being insulted the way she chose to do so? In this context, a syndrome of the post-traumatic stress disorder (PTSD) type developed around the insult, a reaction that was somewhat justified, and the fact that it was an unprovoked assault led to a continual search for "what did I do to deserve this?" accompanied by an attempt (usually futile, as it was in this case) to prove one's own contributory innocence. The trauma is often about being an innocent victim who is wrongly insulted/mistreated, and the PTSD element clinically involves thinking an event through over and over again and wishing that one could get over his/her recurrent rage reaction, repeating itself as a form of reverberating personal lack of forgiveness for this unprovoked attack on one's sensibilities. As Chancer says, "Sadomasochistic dynamics are reproduced so very insidiously, as we come to attack ourselves and each other over and over again. One ethnic group hates another group or an ethnic race, a given class or race oppresses others within it by gender . . . so we may take it out on them in a host of small ways."[3]

Another answer to solving many marital problems founded in sadomasochism involves voluntary freely given altruism and empathy. However, in some relationships, marriage especially, altruism is often, but should not be, the equivalent of masochistic self-abnegation.

In a general way, in a marriage each significant relational interaction needs to be put under a microscope, and the primary mover needs to look at his or her motivation for such and such a thought/action and determine if the marriage's interests are being best served and hopefully will be the interests of both members of the dyad. Then the possible provocateur needs to be identified to determine empathically how the target, the other person in the relationship, has been provoked and is responding and, if a negative response is likely happening, what preventive is indicated and/or what change of course might be warranted.

If you tell someone whom you know likes or loves you that you can't see him or her for a while, you need to determine if this person interprets that remark as being for a few hours or forever, and the best way to do this is to ask the other person to explain exactly what he or she has in mind. This involves being alert on all occasions to how the other person is interacting with you without making assumptions and letting potentially hurtful insults pass through, unidentified and unaddressed. Not only will your concern be appreciated, but misunderstandings can be corrected before they have materialized and hopefully even before they have metastasized. If you say something you regret, it may be that you just misspoke, but if your intent was sadomasochistic ("I am going to bed to avoid seeing you again because of what you just did") and you really said what was on your mind and it was hurtful, then you should correct things as soon as possible, if possible. It is rarely okay to be hurtful even if you so wish it, but certainly if you don't and you are doing so inadvertently, then a red flag should fly about the relational danger of your remark(s) and the possibility that one or more of your interactions will add to the injustices that are being accumulated and may eventuate in really hard feelings that result in your relationship being weighed in the balance, found wanting, and abandoned. Subtle rejection, control, and competitiveness are issues that often need immediate (emergency) recognition, and therefore preventive/corrective measures need to be taken beyond mere observation and acknowledgment of the reality.

Paradoxically, members of a dyad should also be alert to the possibility of excessive closeness.

Mostly, sadomasochistic-based thought changes normal reality-based thinking only very slightly from the natural thinking processes of us all, but you still need to be alert if the content of what you say seems to involve excess (e.g., a secret but powerful idée fixe about punishing the other person for forbidden unacceptable [sexual/oedipal] desires and aggressions, even those that might not come to fruition). At times a self-punishment alert needs to be actively put into place to mollify or avoid danger to a relationship, such as retaliation for another (others) just to avoid serious damage by being constantly alert to its presence. Those who anticipate danger get there first preventively and avoid potential damage and potential ultimate abandonment. The sadistic superego will need to punish, and the masochistic ego will need to be punished out of an excessive unconscious sense of guilt, with pain distributed both as payment for past and permission for further transgressions, so a realization/warning of what is about to happen should offer itself to take center stage to provide insight as to what might happen next. This is a helpful form of mental movement for assessing the past by reviewing what just happened and integrating the present so that one can preventively influence the future in a positive way.

Too often relationships are presumed to be satisfactory, and little to no care or attention is given to the effect of each person upon the other so that preventing future repetition of old insults takes place. Points of sensitivity should not go unnoticed; spouses should know what the other spouse gets riled up about even if, or just because, the issue is minor; and in unfavorable instances all concerned should do what they can to take preventive/corrective measures.

All this just means that relationships take work; avoiding sadomasochistic interactions takes effort to identify, prevent, and repair self-destructive and other destructive interactions to make certain a relationship you want to last continues on a positive note.

These principles also apply to relationships outside the ones between husband and wife. A father-in-law routinely mentions something about a certain despised ethnic group as soon as he enters this group, one to which his son-in-law belongs and is the only person in the family who belongs to it. For example, upon entering a family gathering the father-in-law announces, gratuitously and with no lead-in, that only 6 percent of people who live in New Jersey are Semites. Why would anyone want to know this? Only because it is ethnic-awareness time and clear to all concerned that the father-in-law is a closeted bigot who is being hurtful to his son-in-law and family not so much by anything he says directly but by the consistency whereby he brings up the topic, literally each time he sees his son-in-law, and does so without exception, even though he admits he is wrong and promises to nip it in the bud the next time.

Set your goals according to what is really important, which to me means things relationally and occupationally more than things recreational or financial, so that developing and maintaining a good, solid, rewarding marital relationship and a good job come first, as they should be the focus of any repairs that need to be promptly made.

In conclusion, in a relationship/marriage a divorce doesn't just come about; it is quietly arranged because of lack of attentiveness to the relationship, allowing minor cumulative sadomasochistic provocations (more the rule than the exception) to each take its cumulative toll on the relationship as a whole. The reasons most often given for any divorce are generally rationalizations. The truth is that there is usually a surfeit of small sadomasochistic things that accumulate. Decide beforehand what you want from a relationship, then take steps to make it happen. Eliminate sadomasochism from the playing field, and likely the relationship game has or will be won, meaning that the marriage will likely survive. Especially if either member of the dyad is a masochist or sadist, the tolerance level will be affected incrementally in a positive way.

Sadomasochism in the workplace/corporate sadomasochism. Sadomasochism is expressed by coming late to work, leaving work early, drinking alcohol at lunch, getting into fights with coworkers about what is who's job, playing computer games instead of working, sending flaming e-mails, enmeshing oneself in pornography during work time, and competition with coworkers with whom one could easily work side by side at different or complementary tasks—if only they were so motivated to work cooperatively. But it seems that just the fact that each business has rules and regulations brings out the worst in the employees who feel that "you, my boss, are trying to tell me how to run my life 9–5." And of course, you are; why should it be any different? It's called being hired.

Emotional disturbances at work often take the form of someone who feels that he/she does not deserve to accomplish much, a fear of success that takes the form of being afraid to show one's kind or talented side.

Seeing the boss as a bully rather than as the way he/she is may be politically correct, seducing fellow rebels into one's adversarial camp, but will likely lead to an unnecessary adversarial relationship with one's job and the higher-ups (e.g., the boss). This can lead to putting down and leaving a perfectly suitable job, which can create an atmosphere where one takes on a very dangerous and often ineffective approach: changing one's job when one should be changing one's on-the-job attitude, the attitude that says "No one can do anything right with a boss like mine. He or she just doesn't appreciate me. I'll find someone who does."

When bosses have emotional problems, the workers, their jobs, and ultimately the whole company can suffer. A cyclothymic boss who has severe mood swings independent of reality who—in other words—feels provoked when there is no provocation forthcoming and has temper tantrums is a helicopter boss who controls with words sometimes in the form of tweets in the middle of the night and is excessively critical of his workers, who can do no right, and is apt to create business failure. Similarly problematical is the presence of too many paranoid workers who are hurtful to management no matter how good and effective it is, running a danger to a business being well run and turning the place chaotic deliberately and intentionally hoping to do damage out of a vendetta that only they fully understand and have created themselves out of flimsy internally conjured-up reality. Saying to a coworker within the boss's earshot that this will be a better place to work when the present boss leaves can be a highly destructive thing to do.

Narcissistic bosses give preference to how others see them over what they are doing for the company. They don't care if the company suffers as much as they care if someone higher up than them looks down upon them and instead of criticizing supports them. According to Chancer it is reasonable to note that "Workers are constantly reminded, 'You're little, we're big.'"[4]

It is important to recognize that a worker's sadomasochism may not be the result of a boss's sadomasochistic input but instead may be the consequences of the worker's own disability: a special unhealthy way of dealing with a doable job, thus turning it into a difficult project, and never learning to live with one's negative feelings by acceptance instead of making things worse than they are now.

Society's generally politically correct acceptance of going through life disliking one's job contributes to a great extent to men and women hating what they do "because the gang wouldn't approve of someone who actually liked what they were doing." If possible, one should not stay on in a less than acceptable job that one could at least theoretically escape; doing so does no one much good.

Minimum wages, of course, should not be accepted as being the nature of the beast when individuals might need to unite so they can demand being paid a fair wage. Of course, asking for too much can be masochistically motivated too if one knows that the business will go broke if too much is being paid out in salaries. Making excessive salary demands can be sadomasochism motivated by and originating in oedipal envy (e.g., of the father who has it all ["he has mother"] while the kids have nothing). Feelings against a parent should not be behind this as they are behind other collective protests.

Sadomasochistic companies. Not all companies are brought down by bad business decisions, social shifts in taste, or the ups and downs of the economy or shifting of consumer spending to, for example, the Internet. Many are brought down by the sadomasochistic individuals who work there, as these companies themselves can in their culture be as sadistic to their workers as the people who work for them are sadistic to and sadomasochistic in and with the place they work (actively making it into what they perceive to be passively that proverbial "terrible place to work"). The company that plans a downsizing and announces it in advance but only in some vaguely defined future, keeping everyone guessing and so on edge, is as sadistic as the key worker who keeps the company on edge or pushes it off the edge by threatening to quit but then staying on and doing or just to do damage. The important remedy here involves empathy and altruism: how would you feel if you were in the position of one of your very own victims? If "bad" is the answer, then changing one's approach is the remedy. No one should be motivated by the wish to make others, including one's boss, feel bad. One might be surprised at how often sadists withhold reassurances when simply one can avoid a lot of suffering by being clear about what is at stake and going to happen in the future. The doctor who tells a patient "you have nothing to worry about" stands in sharp contrast to the doctor who gives a patient a diagnosis and withholds a prognosis, especially a good prognosis, secretly desiring that the patient stew as the doctor withholds the truth. It is unfortunately true that some doctors are in the profession because they are dealing with heartfelt sadism by proclaiming pity for the world by being healers, only they are instead making their patients more anxious by keeping them waiting, sometimes for hours or so at a time, and not giving them information they need to feel better about themselves.

A patient says, "After I single-handedly (given that my research assistant lied to me when she was supposed to complete the task list I gave her and left work to paint her deck while I was in training in another building) got everything in order to pass our audit with flying colors, our boss, Henry, whom I had given way too much credit to, even KNOWING she did this in addition to making a lot of other errors which I had told him about, told my assistant Etta that she was 'extraordinary' and offered her a permanent hospital position (nota bene—mine is only a contract that goes to March). Now Etta, already very odd in personality, has a smug smile on her face, and is doing less than ever, and even doing the little she does defiantly at that."

Ageism and the entire range of bigotries infest almost every workplace. I once heard this boss of mine talk about interviewing new hires, ones who were "nice and young," and I can't imagine this decision about whom to keep on the job between me and her would be any different. "He totally disregarded my input on the quality of her work and went ahead and promoted her, essentially giving no credence at all to my position as her supervisor, never mind the fact that I am a hard worker and have a doctorate. I know—carry on and collect a paycheck, which is better than no paycheck. Damn on my having to be sadomasochistic myself just in order to survive."

This sadistic ageist boss felt that workers over a certain age were necessarily incompetent and too weak and brittle to be employed, both literally (that is, hired) and figuratively (that is, used), as in what was to become one of his favorite phrases, "If used, they would break down."

He equated advancing age with progressive deterioration. He spoke of those workers who were still functioning over the age of 60 with hushed amazement. He said of one, "She is 61 years old but still manages to work." To him, those over 60 were like those under 6: unable to function independently. To negatively stereotype those over 60, he had to make his points selectively, disregarding any evidence that did not fit with his preconceived notions. He particularly had to overlook that the relationship between age and "physical deterioration" (his term) was in reality a variable one and that while some of his workers felt older than their stated age, most of his older workers had the reverse problem: they looked older than they used to look but never felt better in their lives, and as for their life's work, many of them didn't start with a bang that turned into a whimper but instead started with a bud that turned into a blossom.

His negative view of his older workers was so convincing that they began to see themselves in the stereotypical way he saw them. Some became openly demoralized. Others tried to disguise what they were because they became convinced that they were flawed. They did grotesque things to themselves (e.g., to their appearance) in a misguided attempt to be admired and loved. Of course, their attempt to get love failed, because they were trying to please a person who needed to dislike them, and they were trying to please him precisely in that area where he needed to dislike them the most. Any real remedies were doomed to failure, because his negativity was not based on reality but instead was transferential; that is, it was based on his own unresolved problems, with growing older projected outward, so that no amount of improved performance on others' part could even begin to change his mind about the ravages of aging. All this, of course, interfered with his hires' ability to do their work and so had the effect of fulfilling his prophecy for him. There is no mind so capable of being read as the mind of the sadomasochist made up to be hurtful."

Some of the more destructive sadistic bosses instead of supporting or helping workers when they are down pick on them, driving them still further down. They issue orders for them to get up, knowing they are too weak to stand. Bosses tell workers who are depressed to cheer up, not merely because they want the workers cheerful but also to attack them for being gloomy, something they do (without doing anything to relieve the gloom) because they find their gloom annoying.

Some sadistic bosses make no attempt to actively create suffering in others. They are content with obtaining schadenfreude, or pleasure from the suffering of others in the cause of which they supposedly have had no detectable hand. They rejoice when they see power overthrown, beauty fade, and talent dry up. They also gloat when a rival rock group fails, saying aloud and with relish "That's what happens to you when you get big." They celebrate when the boss makes a bad business decision and wrecks him or herself, sometimes even when the boss takes the company and them down with him.

In his personal life a boss liked being a spectator of pain. He enjoyed watching TV pictures of rooftop jumpers, and he spoke many times of the pleasure he could have gotten if the law had allowed him to witness executions. He equally enjoyed seeing others fail on a lesser, more symbolic, level so that when he went to the opera he hoped to hear bad notes, and when he went to concerts he hoped to hear musicianly slips. With glee he spoke of how one popular artist's second record, her sophomore trial, was not as popular as her first and how he loved it when a promising political candidate made a fatal Freudian slip, ending his campaign. This boss's devotion to schadenfreude was a way to make himself feel better about himself because he saw himself as a failure in life compared to others. As he saw it, others' pratfalls put him in a comparatively flattering light and proved an existential point he wanted to make, also to put himself in a more favorable light—a point about the failed pretensions of humankind and comeuppance for the pride that he believed regularly and necessarily went before a fall (which fall he had something to do with).

The more seriously sadomasochistic bosses do not wait for fate to act but instead take matters into their own hands. They gleefully make others suffer, putting them down, kicking them when they are down, hitting them again when they try to get up, and being abusive once more when their victims complain about their mistreatment. They dismiss them with "If you can't stand the heat, then get out of the kitchen," then they call them paranoid for being hypersensitive and suggest that their reaction to the abuse is inappropriate while denying that the abuse itself is excessive.

A sadomasochistic boss hated those he falsely concluded were competing with him. And then he deprived them of what they needed, using his considerable political influence within the corporation (his family was on the board of trustees) to wreak his havoc. Those who were "it" knew they had been targeted when after a conference they found his doodles, scraps of paper on the floor or on his desk, with their names carved (really dug) into them, as if they themselves were being mutilated.

In specific, I describe how what I believe to be a sadomasochistic workforce is currently bringing the Veterans Administration (VA) down and doing so at the expense of the veterans who depend on getting care from this institution. A worker there tells the story of how hours were wasted punishing her for making a minor mistake with paperwork at the VA: she had a vet sign the wrong form, presumably triggering a HIPAA violation although nobody realized what had happened. And no damage occurred from her error.

In my opinion, corporations need fewer troubled sadomasochistic bosses and sadomasochistic workers and more untroubled creative bosses and workers who do the right thing for their company and the people it serves, which of course is the purpose of the company in the first place.

Sadomasochistic workers. Sadomasochism is both a specific dynamic factor in certain occupational inhibitions (specific symptoms), ranging from typist's cramp to emotionally induced repetitive strain injury whereby a worker sloughs off because he can no longer physically use the computer keyboard, and a general cause for suffering among workers. Sadomasochistic workers are self-destructive individuals who look for a way to self-defeat/hurt themselves on the job or not get the job done at all. Of course, many occupations provide workers with a ready-made medium and opportunity for occupational self-destructiveness. These companies virtually beg workers to work below par and arrange for them to suffer from their work by offering them job-related unpleasantness such as odd working hours. The workers themselves make a sadomasochistic career move by selecting a job that hurts them and sticking with it instead of taking another job that would be less painfully unproductive. Or they find a decent job and then handle it in an unhealthy, self-destructive way. Some work below par as they stop short of success by acting out as a way to hurt themselves, either deliberately (consciously) or unconsciously. Some damage their anatomy in ways that range from the more to the less obvious. As for the more obvious, they can have accidents on the floor. If they are the composer Robert Schumann, they can maim their fourth finger in the guise of strengthening it. If they are the composer von Weber, they can accidentally drink a glass of nitric acid to ruin their singing voice. If they are the composer Chausson, they can ride their bicycle into a wall and kill themselves. If they are one of my patients, they can, in preparing for a craft show, pick up a saw and unthinkingly cut off a piece of their thumb. Or they can hurt themselves in less obvious ways. They can damage the part of their anatomy they need most not by bashing their head or cutting off a piece of their thumb but instead by tensing instead of relaxing at the computer keyboard, Reich's "character armor" or, as Reich[5] might put it, that is both why they develop a hand syndrome such as carpal syndrome and why rolfing, which is a method of deep muscle massage intended to serve as physical and emotional "relaxation therapy," sometimes works therapeutically as, according to rumor, it did for some pianists who lost the use of a hand due to an emotionally induced paresis.

A doctor with a self-defeating personality disorder went stale because as a way to self-defeat, he made a pact with himself to not keep up with the advances in his field. Also, when trying to write papers he slowed down at the keyboard both because of the emotionally caused repetitive strain injury his therapists diagnosed and as a way to see to it virtually deliberately that he would become disappointed and exasperated with himself. In like manner, although he was talented and knowledgeable, he rarely spoke in public because of a progressively worsening stage fright he put into place to ensure that he would not get his message across to too many important people. When attending conferences, he made jokes from the back of the room to equally sadomasochistic friends when he should have been acting serious, and he made loud fun of the speakers to those of his associates who sat next to him so that these companions would think him a regular guy with a great sense of humor. It seems as if the only thing he really took seriously was his need to hurt himself by being defiant toward authority/those in charge. Of course, his lack of seriousness and his defiance got back to the head of the department and created bad feelings, earning him a place not at the head of the table but rather at the top of the oncoming downsizing list.

Sadomasochistic writer's block. An unsuccessful writer who felt he was doing the best job he could under the impossible circumstances that prevailed in the literary world in which he lived blamed his lack of success on his problems with publishers and critics to the extent that he thought that realizing his dreams was hopeless. What he failed to realize was that his professional failure was self-created. He acted out sexually and then justified his nightly philandering by saying he was living for the moment and wisely improving his self-image through sexual conquest, as if being a professional, not just a sexual, "conquistador" was itself not a good enough way to maintain/improve that self-image. And he arranged for financial reasons to have to take a demeaning draining night job and get overly involved with it instead of just refusing to accept financial help from his wealthy family, something he turned down due to excessive pride and because of his compulsion to buy things that he did not really want or need just to maintain his lifestyle at the expense of pursuing his professional goals.

A wife known for her narcissism was selfish right up to the moment of truth, when she decided to quit her day job to go into business for herself only, as soon as she was about to sign the final papers, to suddenly become what she envisioned as altruistic but what was in fact a self-destructive maneuver meant to keep herself from self-satisfaction. She decided to keep her day job, convincing herself, which was untrue, that "I want to stay here so that I can be sure to be able to buy my husband the things he always wanted to have but that in the past I was too self-centered to get for him."

Many such sadomasochists subtly rationalize their masochism away. Those with little insight think that they fail because they have no talent or ability, and to back up their contention they call themselves bad names such as philistine, lazy, incompetent, shiftless, and stupid. Many convince themselves that a daily dose of unpleasantness is a good thing for them.

They say to themselves, "It's the unpleasant jobs that do, after all, have a measure of security and come with an excellent retirement plan, and it's good to be future oriented, sacrificing pleasure now by saving it for the future as pleasure to come." But they mean "Instead of enjoying myself now when I can, I will postpone enjoyment until I can't," a rationalization, for it is the bright future they are always waiting for, while in the meantime as an exchange they suffer in a drab job or career because they know the bright future will never come. And that is why they agree to the exchange.

Sexual Attraction

Jones notes that consensual sadomasochism should not be confounded with acts of sexual aggression. Moreover, while sadomasochists seek out pain and humiliation in the context of *love* . . . and sex they do not do so in other situations and dislike simple, unfettered violence.[6]

Kramer says, "The brooding unreachable young man, the rebel without a cause, the neglected younger brother, the sardonic outsider, careening on his spiraling downhill course—what woman can resist his dark appeal? . . . The glum and indecisive intellectual, the bitter and isolated observer of life—constellations of traits that look a good deal like depression serve even in middle age to define a certain sort of fascinating man—to feel the force of a lover's moodiness—have the power to overwhelm every sober consideration."[7]

Some sadomasochists ought to be proud of themselves for being sadomasochistic. Some are usefully creative (modern art), and some are to be commended in hindsight for being on the pathway to developing self-pride in being morally right in that occasional instance when they are right about things while others, again looking back, might legitimately be condemned and punished for being philosophically wrong.

Often positive qualities are mixed in with the negative, meaning that some sadomasochism is an advantaged neurosis, as someone completely defies the basic nature of neurosis by turning it into its mirror image and hence a worthwhile endeavor/career.

MIXED POSITIVE AND NEGATIVE VALUES

Hoarding Tendencies Mixed with Healthy Frugality

Frugality is a good thing in small doses, but if excessive it can be more problematical than otherwise. In saving, the reality (unpleasure) principle (the pension plan) is a principle to be followed, but in hoarding, Freud's unreality principle is distorted (with a vengeance). A basic principle of hoarding is "I shop to forget, then keep things I don't need and keep them now because I might need them someday" ("no matter what I have to suffer through now to hold on to them forever"). Another basic principle of hoarding is a denial of the present comfort of all concerned for illusory future gain, an attitude that lies somewhere between a good intention with positive consequences and a bad idea with a negative outcome. In such cases, typically the reality principle has gone amok due to an excessive fear of what the future might hold; therefore, anxiety seems to be at the root of the problem (with hoarding). A current pleasure is renounced out of fear for future well-being, misquoting Alice, "relinquishing jam today for jam tomorrow," which overlooks one possible and sanguine reality, namely that there can be jam for both days. This self-reassuring self-sacrificial behavior establishes the primary masochistic principle of renouncing pleasure now for a rational (rationalized) reason. But as with many examples of hoarding, the hoarding process itself ensures that tomorrow will be worse, not better, than today, as can happen when a house fills up and has to be declared unlivable. Another sadistic measure in hoarding is failure to consider others in the equation. It is sadomasochistic to continue hoarding anyway knowing that down deep one is being sadistic toward others when, as part of sacrificing present gain for future achievement, the hoarder puts partners, family, and coworkers in harm's way by his or her unnecessary sacrifice for a future gain they know, in spite of the rationalizations, to be either entirely unrealistic to expect or unlikely to in any event come about in a meaningful way.

In one case, a patient hoarded birthday cakes stacked up to the ceiling, all soon having or to become inedible. In another case, a patient saved the knives that had the best reflection so she could check her makeup regularly by looking into the blade to see if she was getting older by the minute.

Hoarding is especially sadistic when a person fills up the house with things nobody really needs and sadistically puts persons out to make room for things of little worth that additionally heap risk upon all concerned (e.g., the risk of the elderly falling while trying to avoid some impediment) or puts the family, including family members who have a full-time job, in the position of having to virtually quit work to come help out, something that is distinctly sadistic because the hoarder knows that he or she is causing hard times for others. Hard times now may only ensure even harder times in the future, especially true for those involved who find themselves caring for others who are unable, no matter what is said or done, to pull themselves out from under the first person's junk collecting.

In the positive aspects of hoarding, masochists make some people's self-importance and self-definition a positive thing for a specific and relatively predictable but valid non–self-punitive purpose (e.g., the butterfly collector).

Another positive aspect of hoarding is that to hoard you have to shop, and this can be rewarding for those who have nothing else to do and not self-punitive for those who with plenty of money spend themselves down to broke just to accumulate things they do not need.

Narcissism Mixed with Charitability

Narcissism is a good thing when there is reason to be narcissistic for purposes of bettering oneself and others as part of the fallout. A doctor is unsuccessful as a practitioner, so he prides himself on knowing what a good teacher he is, helping other doctors practice. He is thinking not only of himself but also of both himself (narcissistic) and his patients (altruistic). Narcissism by itself is a sadomasochistic (bad) thing when it is mostly exclusionary, especially when it is presented as otherwise (e.g., "I don't leave you for me, but I do so for your own good").

Altruism Mixed with Selfishness

The sadomasochist can be the good self-sacrificial altruist when he or she (masochistically) takes others' needs excessively into consideration over his or her own. But too often in sadomasochism the negativity of the intent has the effect of obscuring a positive outcome. Here sadomasochism becomes admirable simply because of the nobility of sacrifice and effort involved, and one can be proud of oneself for the self-abnegation implied and the possibility that hard times for you today will somehow thwart hard times for you/someone else tomorrow. A woman about to die of alcoholism leaves the care of her four dogs to a friend who graciously (altruistically) accepts the challenge but does nothing to stop the process even though she knows very well what is going to happen next, because as soon as she can she is going to give the dogs up to the shelter for adoption.

Love Mixed with Hatred

Sadomasochism is an essential part of love ("I'd like to squeeze you to death") and creates in some instances lasting relationships, especially when self-sacrifice is for the true benefit of someone else. Too often, however, love dies when the lover recognizes the hardship caused to him or her via the self-sacrifice involved and, becoming tired and reasonably selfish, wishes to discontinue the relationship based on altruism of his or her own, himself benefiting.

Nonsadomasochistic love is true positivity, not true negativity otherwise rationalized as being its opposite (positivity). Sadomasochism can involve the promise of care for others, hiding the true motivation of total lack of concern for others disguised as charity, that consists of an uncharitable charitable lack of concern for oneself.

Predictability Mixed with Uncertainty

Sadomasochists can consciously choose being sadomasochistic, then call it a compulsion because they know they are getting something they want for themselves at others' expense and are ashamed of that, or they can be highly principled, their sadomasochism being a personal form of honest expression whereby others soon come to learn and know what they can count on—although admittedly the principles, though predictable, themselves can be somewhat or close to dysfunctional or immoral and potentially destructive to self and others. It is this core sadomasochist who is so unpredictable that we never know what to expect from him or her.

Perfectionism Mixed with Carelessness

The perfectionist's goals may involve doing things philosophically absolutely right not as a hidden expression of the need for control of the deviant other (who is presumably doing everything wrong) and not so as a way to bring others up short as defective (due to criticizing them by implication for being imperfect) but instead as central to recommending that all concerned live to fulfill a certifiable valid ultimate achievement.

Omniscience Mixed with Uncertainty

Sadomasochistic omniscience may involve controlling people based on the assumption of being able to do so because one is always right and holds suitable and justified power in terms of one's goals. A sadomasochist may in fact know it all and what is best for all under most or all circumstances. Omniscient sadomasochists may know what is right and simultaneously insist that others follow their dictates and always go along with them. This works but only when what is at stake is widespread presumptuousness that covers the right thing. Sadomasochistic omnipotence can also be a good quality when it provides leadership worth following, at which point a group might do well to relinquish its own lines of independent thought to follow an even greater power and control as well as functionality by being guided by a sadomasochistic omniscient guru.

There are good sadomasochistic individuals who have an inborn talent for leadership, often one that cannot be taught, such as the power to hypnotize other people. But there is a thin line between organizational abilities and the omniscient sense of an irrational, inflexible certainty of purpose and unquestionable knowledge of others' minds made up not for good but instead for some arbitrary need for control of others in a hurtful way. Thus, the steadfast omniscient "I know better than you" individual can be a reliable chief out to conquer as the worthy benign guru there to force others to rally around, being one who can protect/influence others when others do in fact need guidance because they have gotten out of line—the guru not out to control but rather to lead. In some cases this can be a good thing, even when he or she is being arbitrary but for that reason alone is still able to provide superficially valid approaches to solving bad problems, offering us seeming immovable platforms in space (a fixed position one can count on to always be there as a solid rock, one to reason and act from and return to whenever necessary), helping those who may be floundering to instead establish a sensible, doable, creative, workable temporary or lifetime plan for themselves and/or beloved others based on concrete principles of effective guidance instituted by those who give that guidance rationally, who are in the know mainly out to unselfishly benefit others by lending them their insight and offering to share their power yet are aware of when to retreat strategically, perhaps after having gone too far arbitrarily. In this one sense sadomasochism is yesterday's cruelty to self and others that may very well turn out to be today's plan for a happy tomorrow—the goal that turns into a happy plan for today.

Controlling Tendencies Mixed with Passivity

Some sadomasochists as controlling people compulsively set helpfully firm, if excessively arbitrary, limits on others making it certain that others are under their control, giving others a good plan to follow while not depriving them of current pleasures to which they are entitled or disrupting current admirable achievements. A sadomasochistic mother hurtful to her family's functionality and creativity complains that her daughter, who is far into adulthood, still insists on driving to the supermarket to pick up some of the blue potato chips she likes when in fact her mother has provided the party she is giving with some other chips that ought to be good enough for anybody. The mother is a sadist, but the daughter, although she yearns to rebel and has her rights too, is also learning rational discipline.

Morality Mixed with Amorality

It is not sadomasochistic when the potential for positive accomplishment is taken into account when issuing edicts or advocating behaviors that have less of an emotional and more of a theoretically valid basis, one with a realistic bent. But destroying a restaurant because the owner has the wrong sociopolitical orientation, according at least to those with an opposing point of view, can be sadomasochism on a seriously invalid basis.

Taking sides is not sadomasochistic when it involves forcefully aligning with a person because he or she is right, but it is sadistic when it involves siding with a person just to (unsupportively) take sides regardless of intellectual correctness and moral justification.

The relative nature of selfishness means that in evaluating that and its opposite, selflessness, one can see these things from the viewpoint of the well-being of all concerned, not so that individual interests conflict with universal values constituting a rational philosophy.

Workaholism Mixed with Laziness

There is at times little distinction between a strong work ethic and sadomasochism manifest in refusing to take a vacation for oneself, which can be hurtful to oneself (and possibly others in one's family). At what point on the continuum is it sadomasochistic to refuse to take time off even though one's spouse asks you to travel, but you complain that relaxing takes time overall out of your work schedule? It is certainly sadomasochistic for a company that is part of a merger to take a worker's pension or vacation time away from him or her, touting the traditional rule that now that you are promoted to management and management is unpaid for overtime, you get your straight salary and no more.

Honesty Mixed with Attitude/Image

If others are going to hate and punish you, they should at least hate you for what you truly are rather than for what you make yourself out to be.

Withholding (Permission) Mixed with Ambivalence about What Is the Right Way to Do Things

Sadomasochistic withholding can take the form of teasing and not delivering things promised as being forthcoming. This is not always a negative virtue. Positive virtues of this manifestation of sadomasochistic behavior include indecisiveness that staves off the premature implementation of bad ideas and bad decisions and indicates the presence of a degree of the responsibility to all concerned that can be provided/enhanced by delay. But we are dealing with sadomasochism when a refusal to yield is arbitrary and based on a philosophy that is autistic, arbitrary, and presumptuous, mainly involving a refusal to budge.

Vacillating Mixed with Absolute Certainty

Vacillating is not sadomasochistic when it involves taking precautions when there is no aggression and/or hostile vacillation (consisting of nonstop seeing all sides of an issue) intended. This can overall be more perspicacious than paralytic as long as it contributes to the healthful evolutionary growth of the functionality of all concerned. Sometimes constantly changing one's mind is a sign of weakness; sometimes constantly changing one's mind is a sign of strength (carefulness and consideration). There are victories and Pyrrhic victories.

In many cases, however, delaying the implementation of bad decisions is a virtue of doubting however sadomasochistic it might at first appear to be, for people who doubt can help themselves and others avoid making serious and sometimes fatal mistakes that would be the product of excessive impulsivity and premature activity.

Vacillation is highly sadomasochistic when it takes the form of teasing others by being too open-minded, seeing all points of view not in the service of giving time and putting effort into developing understanding but instead in the service of stalling by indecisiveness.

Doubting sadomasochists can protect others from uncertainty or torture others with their uncertainty. A sadomasochistic inpatient constantly brooded about "Did I bump you?" That is, he wondered if he had bumped into someone to whom he had gotten too physically close. To ask his question, he had to come close so that the person he was directing his apologies to could hear him without uncertainty. Alas, being heard virtually ensured that he would bump into his victim, at which point he had to ask once again "Did I bump you?" This behavior on his part was so intolerable to others that ultimately he had to be locked up in the seclusion room to prevent him from being so intrusive that others couldn't live their lives or do their work at all. For this individual, the positive virtues attached to his obsessive bumping questions involved him feeling involved with an audience and an integral part of the group of those he was in fact victimizing.

Expressed Hostility Mixed with Controlled Hostility

Sadomasochism can involve a passive-aggressive attack or can reflect a protective sensible cautiousness on those fronts where impulsivity, the obverse of slowness and stickiness, is more the enemy.

Punctiliousness Mixed with Unreliability

Being on time is a positive virtue and can be even more so when the individual pushes all concerned too hard not to be late (e.g., he or she runs across subway platforms to catch the express train on the adjacent platform, breathless as he or she may become, in the meantime courting the danger of tripping and/or knocking other people over or having an asthma attack). Here being punctilious may involve being sensibly reliable, as it takes the valuable form of being highly motivated to give the other person—say, the one waiting—what he or she can count on. But when pushed to excess, punctiliousness can cause the nonpunctilious other person great emotional or physical discomfort, and demands to be on time cause the person waiting a great sense of guilt for being just a minute or two delayed. Punctiliousness is especially irritating/unsettling if a person sets a time for meeting then after getting there early thinks that the other person is late.

In sum, punctiliousness can be a positive feature of sadomasochism or can create one of its unwanted, unpleasant, unworkable, interpersonal annoying manifestations.

Wearisomeness and Lack of Confidence Mixed with Confidence/Overconfidence

Worrisomeness is hurtfully sadomasochistic when it amounts to unproductive fidgeting and fretting about minor issues but healthfully nonsadomasochistic when it provides the basis for lifesaving prompt/early interventions, for example, by suggesting that a patient get a second medical opinion in cases of an underdiagnosed or improperly diagnosed malady.

Also to be on the lookout for is pseudosadomasochistic or healthfully sadomasochistic worrisomeness meant for personal reassurance that turns out to be an anxiety reducer for the first party though at the expense of bringing further anxiety to the second party.

Preconceived Notion and Argumentativeness Mixed with Uncertainty

Stubbornness and argumentativeness (however much it lacks consideration for others' points of view) can enhance functionality for those people whose opposition is simultaneously powerful but misguided. This is sanguine behavior, not sadistic obstinacy, and does not seriously raise the question of how to tell sadomasochism from virtuous input when it involves activity that knowingly prevents one from succumbing to charlatans, facilitates not hinders a useful social activity, or otherwise helps individuals avoid yielding to something that he or she should instead stubbornly resist. Clearly, sadomasochism is profitably mainly identifiable by intent (motivation), which is difficult to determine, especially since there is so often a mixture of motivations. Resisting opposition from a child, for example, can ultimately speak favorably to the child's future, as when a parent demands (by withholding tuition) that a child go to law school when the child indulges him or herself by going to art school in pursuit of a profession that he or she is unlikely to be successful at. Accusations of parental sadomasochism are often present here but can be unfair, and it is the accuser who is being sadomasochistic in the service of so-called being true and helpful to all concerned under the often impractical guise of "only doing what you love."

There is a balance between giving good advice and acting out the desire to control another that is on a continuum, and this balance is not always easy to achieve. The child may at first complain, then only later see what at first appeared to be sadomasochistic pressure from the parent as in fact the parent doing and saying things for the child's ultimate good and best interests. I myself spent too much liberal arts time analyzing Bach fugues and excitedly identifying the rain motive in Wagner's *Die Valkyrie,* a current pleasure that seemed to have a purpose at the time but had no future to it at all, and I was doing other liberal arts things that trained me for nothing marketable (and I embarked on this program even against my parents' well-considered advice, as if they were being cruelly uninformed to insist that I go to medical school, which I fortunately did). I was doing what I loved, but it didn't in any way love me back. However, we only hear of the cases where the artist-to-be thus pushed ignored the parent's wishes and became a famous artist or composer. And we rarely hear of the cases where the artist ignored the parent's advice and truly became "a starving artist" not necessarily in the good romantic sense of the term but rather in the venue of having nothing to eat.

Rebelliousness Mixed with Consideration for Others

Too often, social sentiment guides us sadomasochistically by taking the side of the rebellious child who knows his or her own mind but not his or her own talent. On the other hand, the child who says "I gave myself the summer off" by refusing to take a temporary job in a hardware store as a salesperson to help needy parents involves a child who is sadomasochistically being inconsiderate of the parents and their budget and being sadomasochistic by offering nothing but disregard for the parents' financial needs, so that while "doing his/her own thing" the child is hurting the parents who also have their own things they want and need to do. In those families where an extramarital affair is blessed as having proved profoundly beneficial and saved the relationship, all objects in the affair should be considered and their feelings and needs taken into account before the relationship is considered "saved by the cheating."

Excessive Obsessive Dysfunctional Morality Mixed with Iconoclasm

Empty torturing of others, often by enforcing rigid moral percepts in the form of harsh rules and regulations rigidly imposed in preparation for installing further sadomasochistic precautions, can on the bright side spin off regulations that encourage (force) others to get certain things of an admirable (though strictly theoretical) nature done. But on the harsh side it can also pain others by insisting that they do rituals that are totally foreign to them and unproductive for most people in the (for them) real world. For example, we have the moral injunction involving "take off your shoes before you enter my apartment so that you don't bring in dirt that scratches my new linoleum floors," when this in a rental property where tenants come and go with dirty shoes no matter what the rules and regulations are.

In conclusion, in my opinion, lack of consideration is on the low (less serious) end of the sadomasochistic spectrum that starts on top with inconsideration and goes all the way to the bottom to murder. Even the best qualities of sadomasochism can still hurt feelings and sadistically break hearts, though the intent is admirable and the results even somewhat acceptable.

5

The Fundamental Role That Anger Plays in Individual Sadomasochism

Anger and the divisiveness it produces play a core role in masochistic and sadistic individuals and groups. Due to anger, all involved run the risk of dissolving into splintered individuals and groups, leading to a solitary existence, or, as happened with the psychoanalytic movement, rival non- or anti-Freudian believers ultimately forming ideological subtypes. These subtypes still exist today based on different foci clung to dramatically without integrating the various possibilities into one overarching philosophy such that some psychoanalytic groups focus on the there and then and insist upon pure theories of causative oedipal rivalry, while other psychoanalytic groups focus on the here and now, insisting on current (interpersonal) events as being the important formative ones. The possibility that many formative trends account for the final outcome does not admit itself into a comprehensive theory that goes beyond description of how each subgroup struggles to the death for theoretical primacy. Individual identity not only creates but also emerges from and is intensified by one's "group affiliation," that is, not "I am a mental health worker" but rather "I am a Freudian." Group formation serves to hide but not explain individual motivation and subdue the self-questioning guilt that can go along with it. Thus, "I am not paranoid, or homicidal, I am just influenced by my group and its ideals about who is and who isn't right."

THREE CORE QUESTIONS ABOUT ANGER AND SADOMASOCHISM

I believe it is worthwhile viewing sadomasochism from the viewpoint of Freud's tripartite model of psychological illness, so in the following discussion I explore the validity of breaking sadomasochistic activity into the familiar components of id, superego, ego ideal, and ego, meaning that like many patients with a personality disorder, sadomasochists have a problem with anger and guilt and an inability to incorporate their anger healthfully into their psychological functioning, hence the title of the excellent paper by Inbar, Ariely, Pizarro, and Gilovich: "Moral Masochism: On the Connection between Guilt and Self-Punishment."[1] (This title also suggests that sexual masochism will not be the focus of the following discussion.)

The answers to three core questions about hostility and sadomasochism help us recognize and make a dynamic, and hence more accurate, diagnosis of sadomasochism. I pose and attempt to answer these three core questions, because the answers to them help define a core aspect of sadomasochistic personality disorder, possibly once again making it an officially recognized personality disorder, one that I hope will reappear in any forthcoming *DSM-6*. The questions and their answers all emphasize the underlying (suppressed) hostility that is at the heart of this syndrome. These questions are:

1. Why do sadomasochists get so angry? (The answer goes to determining the specific anger triggers that release the characteristic sadomasochistic angry response, such as humiliation.)
2. Why can't (or won't) sadomasochists express their anger directly? (The answer goes to why, as Potter-Efron and Potter-Efron, state in another context, sadomasochists rarely view "anger as an enemy, something to avoid at all costs,"[2] but welcome its expression as good for a relationship or even good for the soul, that is, the state of one's mental health).
3. How exactly do sadomasochists express what relatively little anger they can if not muster then at least feel it is worthwhile for them to reveal?

The answers here go into making up the specific anger styles that sadomasochists select to express how angry they feel, however indirectly (physically and morally) they express their feelings, ranging from annoyance to rage at their targets of physical and mental brutality.

The questions themselves along with their answers tell us not only much about the structure of this mental disorder but also about how to help many of those it afflicts. We learn of ways to deal effectively with the submerged hostility that exists behind what appears to be the neutral to pleasant sadomasochistic facade some sadomasochists manifest, at least when they are on their best behavior, a facade that often contradicts actual motivated behavior (e.g., consisting of refusing to support a spouse emotionally though he or she is correct about something and has done nothing wrong, the typical mother-in-law triad that leads to so many hard feelings between otherwise sensible people).

Sadomasochism is, however, not strictly about anger; rather, libidinal factors get into the mix too and are, as the psychoanalyst might say, fused with the anger. Sadomasochists, perhaps more than any other patients, fuse their anger with their libidinal desires, leading to a strong connection between emotional pain and hurting all concerned physically and mentally, as pain, anger, and sexuality are meshed/transformed into one package. This can present emotionally (as pertains with moral masochism/moral sadism) or physically (as with a paraphilia in action), typically the whipping or spanking often associated with sadomasochism.

As examples, passive-aggressive sadomasochism and paranoid sadomasochism exemplify the relationship between anger and sadomasochism.

Passive-Aggressive Anger and Sadomasochism

Sadomasochists, in contradistinction to many other individuals with a personality disorder, such as those suffering from passive-dependency or passive-aggressiveness, suppress their anger feelings only to later come to express them, at least most of the time, obliquely (and only, and on rare occasions, directly). This oblique expression of anger, masochistic toward oneself and sadistic to others, generally occurs in the context of chronic hostility. Rarely associated with a specific single grievance, oblique anger frequently requires no immediate provocation. In fact, the mechanism of deflection may break down in the face of direct provocation that, by acting as an especially potent trigger, opens the way to more overt (direct) forms of expression of anger.

The most typical examples of oblique hostile expressions of anger in the guise of sadomasochism are those that contain significant passive-aggressive components such as those relating to moralizing. These include preaching at others purportedly, but not actually, for others' own good; excusing oneself by accusing others, thus making others feel guilty when the fault is one's own; killing with kindness, being overly nice to one's purported adversaries as a way to hurt them by making them feel guilty (a variety of the Midas punishment whereby the sadomasochistic individual acts sadomasochistic by turning a positive gesture into a vehicle for a negative one, as did the sadistic patient who along with a Christmas card sent a letter detailing his complaints against the recipient—speaking of improving relations by airing legitimate grievances); and bumbling behaviors in which an otherwise competent or well-coordinated person becomes ineffective (e.g., less than useful or actually harmful to another individual or to society as a whole). In the same category but more specifically sadomasochistically retaliatory are the actions of the patient who punished his therapist for the hypocrisy of demanding money in return for imparting understanding by paying his therapy bill in meager installments, as it were, slowly starving the doctor; the obsessional sadomasochistic student who, angered by his teacher, responded not with a tirade but instead with a long incomprehensible essay that, he gloated, "made her writhe to read it"; the wife who replied to her husband's boast that a painting he bought many years ago for $1,000 was now worth 50 times that amount by reminding him of the many similar bargains he had turned down over the same period and noting that in fact the painting was in an early style that the market had subsequently disowned; and the boss who, when displeased with an employee, would announce, "I have a bone to pick with you," then keeps the employee in suspense until a meeting took place, one that the boss deliberately scheduled to be a few nervous-making weeks away.

A friend says of her son:

> Don has been facing some crap at work in the small law firm he is in, and I told him he has to start drawing some personal boundaries if he ever wants to be taken seriously. Fred, his father, was a "good guy" too; in fact, everyone loved him, but he also got walked all over at work and never got any promotions. I wish Don would be more like me in that department, as I really have no trouble at all pushing back when the situation requires it.
>
> For one, the man who owns the practice had promised him a raise a few weeks ago but smelled of beer when he did so and then forgot about it. Now he put a woman in charge of the practice and she told Don that SHE is now in charge of the raises, and he is not getting one because even though he is a hard worker and knows a lot about the law, he lacks "common sense" and she feels that maybe this job is not right for him. She also told him he should grow a beard so he can look more assertive in court. WOULD ANY OF THAT KIND OF TALK BE ACCEPTABLE IF IT WAS A MAN BOSS TALKING TO A FEMALE SUBORDINATE? He is very discouraged, and I told him to start looking for another position. He works till 7:00 p.m. every night and goes in on weekends and only makes $48,000. What a winning profession.

In this category too is the man who was undergoing therapy three times a week and expressed his anger at his psychiatrist for taking an annual one-month vacation by resuming sessions with a former psychiatrist whom he had left some months before, even though the patient didn't really need the interim support and himself recognized that seeking it was actually counterproductive due to introducing an element of complicating uncertainty into the process. (Note that the degree of self-harm varies here from one example to another.)

Sadomasochistic passive-aggressive anger may consist of anger expressed by *omission,* anger expressed by *commission,* or both. Either form of expression may be justified by error or lofty motives, for both make a perfect cover for secret malicious intent.

Among sins of *omission* (justified by unintentional error) are forgetting (commonly an anniversary) and Freudian slips involving such behavior as not hearing or overlooking.

An example of a sin of *commission* is verbal accident-proneness, one form of which is another classical Freudian slip behavior where one says the consciously unwanted thing because one fails to perceive one's (negative) motivating attitude, perceives it too late, or mistakenly believes that attitude to have been concealable, with the individual remaining unaware of the implications of his or her actions or words until awareness comes, only not in enough time. Thus, a psychiatrist, thanking his supervisor for helping him with an article he was writing, failed to recognize the secret death wish expressed when, his tongue slipping, he told the senior person, "I will be thankful to you until the day *you* die" (my emphasis). Of interest here is the overlap between indirect expression of anger in a passive-aggressive fashion and commission of unethical deeds that are intended to be possibly amoral and rely for the impact of the anger on defying socially accepted moral standards, such as those that involve flag burning or keeping fledgling wild birds in an indoor cage.

Sins of commission are typically justified by lofty motives. These include lack of concerns for the material, moral, or psychological interest/well-being of the victim and/or society. Recently there have been episodes of refusing to stand up during the playing of the National Anthem, whereby actions are both purportedly meant to exercise the right to protect one's freedom of speech and personal expression and also become sadistic not so much for themselves but due to the venue or context in which a right is discharged specifically in a way that is hurtful to the rights (wishes) of others. A sadomasochistic subject might give disappointing gifts that, however, embody moral or aesthetic values compatible with benevolent intentions and dispense advice morally/theoretically unimpeachable but consciously or unconsciously clearly meant to have hurtful implications, such as calling an author's attention to a trivial typo found in an already published manuscript so that you, the author, can profit by not making the same mistake again. In the latter case this may or may not involve truly constructive criticism, depending on motivation, which is hard to discern.

Is the informer trying to cast aspersions on what happened the last time or trying to forestall the same thing from happening the next time, or is this just hateful sadistic behavior meant to put a given individual down, clearly not meant to be a helpfully instructive teaching experience, since the circumstances provide no good opportunity for being corrective. Other examples include pointing out that an author used the term "symptomatology" rather than "symptom," called to the author's attention seemingly less to teach than to criticize, and advice given to commit fraud by not reporting a repeat dog bite to one's insurance company because this exposes the dog to being euthanized should there have been or should there be a second (or in this case fifth) bite.

Typical of sadomasochists is the refusal to take any responsibility for their deviant behavior. A colleague of mine objected to my use of the term "patient" if I used it to refer to those who were not actually in treatment with me. I looked up the term in a medical dictionary and found that my usage was correct, consistent with one of two formal definitions of the term the dictionary suggested. My colleague's reply to what I thought to be helpful advice said, "I am going to continue to do it my way nevertheless."

Paranoia, Anger, and Sadomasochism

The intensity of blame of others along with self-absolution turns one from she who attacks another to he who is attacked, characteristic of individual and group paranoia. Marked rivalry is characterized by rivalry, resentment, and blame shifting as part of the sadomasochistic attitude and motivation for simple or elaborate sadomasochistic thought and action. Heated political discussions/battles meant to clarify matters or reach compromise have about the same lack of effect as trying to talk a patient of mine out of the delusion that he has swallowed a cat and needs emergency abdominal surgery to remove it.

In a subtle way, sadomasochistic patients, who may be psychotic, are frequently unpredictable: they are openly charming until one does something they consider to be wrong, at which point they snap, leaving the other member of the dyad completely mystified about what happened but certain that he or she did something awful. Based on several cases of mine, I learned that people who talk to frogs sitting on mushrooms or tutelaries floating about are full of relational traps, and it is virtually impossible not to fall into one or more of them and to never quite know what one did, if dumped, to deserve being gotten rid of. They set the process going by some impulsive provocative behavior on their part; the other person reacts negatively, then this other person accuses the first party of overreacting and being the cause of the whole thing. A man is telling another man about the content of a television show. The listener expresses his disagreement. The first man snaps, "I'm not saying that, they are," and the relationship deteriorates from there. Some of the worst and most dangerous sadomasochists are professors who give bad grades over philosophical differences, ruining careers. Sometimes being the victim of sadomasochism is just a matter of bad luck in getting the wrong professor assignment. A professor savaged a student for misdiagnosing hysteria as schizophrenia and virtually ruined his career this way; later the student, now himself a professor, saw a series of patients this first doctor misdiagnosed, and the problem turned out to be one in reverse: that is, all these patients were schizophrenic, but she misdiagnosed all of them as hysterical.

The clinical manifestations of anger in both masochism and sadism can be overt or subtle, in the latter case like schadenfreude. Both individuals and groups brag/complain whereby the central issue becomes "how I am being treated" and "my annoyance with you for not treating me better is mounting, and anyway who do you think you are and what do you think you can get away with?" (the status of being angry with someone else confers status upon the one who is angry for being the one on top and the joy of not this time being the underdog/victim); reactive antialtruism based on reaction formation against empathy deemed excessive ("you are draining me dry with all your demands and neediness") or inadequate; active versus passive enjoyment, such as "It's me who deserves to treat you meanly because you provoked me to do so, and it's you who wants to be treated angrily otherwise you wouldn't be so provocative"; sexual and nonsexual displays depending on the issue/people involved; biting cruelty ranging from nagging to yelling to becoming physically violent; various and often random negative accusations both true and possibly exaggerated/paranoid; false accusations, including those that imply or are easily misinterpreted as implying accusations of (evil) criminal intent; deprecation of oneself and or another although another one is doing one's best; issues related to martyrdom, which is mostly anger at oneself for being insufficiently self-sacrificial accompanied by deferential feelings to another (who is sadistically given the privilege to do the dirty work of self-sacrifice when it comes to you as victim); and a tendency to be oral (bite), to control (sully), and to dominate (in the vernacular crudely but accurately put as b*ll-busting and c*ck teasing), doing a routine pecker-check, and blaming others for things one is oneself responsible for (done in a paranoid fashion) should a serious screwup be detected. In my case a cousin kept complaining that there was something wrong with my e-mail, though the problem was with her iPad.

Tweeting and spouting things later regretted and speaking foolishly are in great measure products of the loss of control of one's anger that is a significant element in the structure of aspects of sadomasochism. This is in part due to the horror of a vacuum, for in a vacuum anxiety and other unpleasant feelings tend to break through, since there is no resistance, and escalate to fill up the feeling of emptiness, making things ultimately worse.

Because this anger may not show up in its original form (mostly it is kept civilized and expressed passive-aggressively), one goal is to help the anxious sadomasochist relax from the very beginning. Suggesting worried sadomasochists stop overreacting and worrying about every little thing can work—should the individual in question be effectively helped to identify with the relaxed therapist instead of perceiving the advice as a command—a command as something that the sadomasochist, like any "good sadomasochist," can't or won't follow.

I get the impression that on average sadomasochistic individuals who are also depressed tend to be angrier than people who are not additionally depressed. This is partially explainable on a causal basis, because the anger of depression is synergistic with the anger of sadomasochism. It follows that some depressed men and women take their angry/violent feelings and fantasies out on themselves to create their own suffering and that this takes the form of lowered self-esteem, suicidal tendencies, or suicidal behavior, all of which walk things back to intensify their original anger. Indeed, depression is little more than self-directed sadomasochism, and sadomasochism is in part other-directed depression. One can take their angry/violent feelings and fantasies out on the world, causing many others to suffer, doing so either passive-aggressively or openly in the form of verbal temper tantrums or physical abuse of others. Or one can be paranoid: with paranoia being little more than sadomasochism directed from the self and at the world. Many individuals are both depressed and paranoid, as was the man who blew up his own house to get back at his wife for winning money and the house in a divorce settlement, injuring her emotionally, injuring passers-by emotionally and physically, and hurting himself seriously in the process. Paranoid attacks on others are often the core of individual or group violence and come with a degree of justification that is not warranted, leading to blood in the streets.

A common denominator is that angry sadomasochistic individuals desire to create misery in others. As Oldham and Morris say, "remember that interactions with sadistic individuals are no win situations."[3] They want to spread the pain around, so they attempt to dominate, control, and castrate others. They might do this to have company in their misery; they punish others in a way that resembles how they themselves feel dominated, controlled, and castrated. Or they might wish to elevate a flagging self-esteem or to repair a mangled masculine or feminine self-image by being the tyrant instead of the one tyrannized or the castrator instead of the one being castrated (ambushed). A man appealed to all his friends to tell him what to do to feel less angry precisely so he could reject all their suggestions as unhelpful, inadequate, and hopelessly outdated. As he once admitted to me during a therapeutic hour, "My annoying impossible depression is a way to be as angry with others and make others as angry with me, as I feel angry with myself."

Sadomasochism is a defensive way to hide anger under the guise of giving or receiving pain retaliatively. Both masochists and sadists are too highly attuned for their own good to other people's negative attitudes about anger issues, especially the attitude of partners who even hint they are feeling angry. Masochists and sadists find even a normal degree of annoyance to be appalling and threaten to dislike, criticize, and abandon others out of retaliation consisting of angry feelings of their own.

Additionally, sadomasochism already in place creates anger as well as the other way around. A sadomasochistic temperament is an important component in a person's *anschauung* and hence sadomasochistic thought and behavior.

Here is an example of the clinical manifestations of temperament: I asked a ticket master for a round-trip ticket to New York's Penn Station. He railed at me for being repetitious because there is only one station in New York, and hence I was wasting his and my time by being redundant.

Others' tolerance of anger is also a factor. One partner doesn't mind being abused, for he just sees anger as a normal emotion. For another, a relationship full of anger is no longer viable.

LOW SELF-ESTEEM

Anger and self-image often are related to each other. Masochists are often nice guys, and sadomasochists are often "difficult people." Masochists want most of all to see themselves and be seen as good people; to suffer and be seen as suffering is good, while to be happy is bad. Sadists often like to project an image of being nasty. Why else would the ticket taker not just simply answer my question? It gives them a sense of power and triumph when they have very little else in their lives to make them feel both good and important.

A clinical manifestation characteristic of sadomasochistic men and women is that though they look full of self-pride, they basically suffer from low self-esteem, which guides them on their interpersonally distortive ways. Who else would want to self-defeat other than someone who has few positive feelings about him or herself?

Pure and simple, sadomasochists are angry with themselves and others and to a notable and often unhealthy degree. Those with low self-esteem often denigrate others as they do themselves.

Self-esteem is often low in sadomasochists because of a range of specific negative feelings about oneself. These negative feelings and the resultant lowering of self-esteem are attributable to:

- A faltering view along the lines of "nobody hates me like I do" (giving one a special position in life);
- Self-punishment for having been/feeling mistreated;
- Compulsively seeking failure because they believe that failure is all they realistically are entitled to;
- Finding themselves indulging in excessive self-sacrifice;
- Sexual and occupational problems such as impotence (e.g., during the performance of paraphiliac sexual acts and creative block due to work-related inhibitions);
- Allowing themselves to gladly suffer from humiliating paraphilias. Some become pedophiliac because they question their value as adults. They select children for sexual encounters because they themselves can only relate fearlessly to someone dependent, helpless, small, and too weak to protest, complain, or fight back and so too needy and scared to break away and leave.
- Having become rough-trade paraphiliacs who feel entranced only by people they consider to be lowlife, as they favor people whom they can view as being beneath them over those they view as their equals or superiors. They become attracted to such people only because they do not feel entitled to seek people on their own level, only people such as desperate losers, the sole ones they feel whose attention they can get in the first place and will command, those they feel worthy of. Some are so sadomasochistic that as prostitutes after the act is over they don't even accept the money they are in fact owed but instead claim that they have sex out of love or due to the wish to humiliate a client. Often it is the outcome of child abuse that shows here. In one case, the child abuse consisted of being devalued for being a change-of-life baby, as if the timing of when the person was born had some special relevance to one's basic value.
- The feeling, correct or not, of being currently hated, rejected, or disdained by sadists whose negative evaluations are both imagined or there in reality and being allowed to rule. This is particularly painful when the hating sadists are one's own children who have decided now that since they have families of their own and don't need the support of mom and dad, it's time to get back at their parents for all the things they did wrong by ignoring them more or less completely. In one case one of the children demanded that his mother enumerate all the bad

things she did to him three times exactly before he would ever speak to her again. Sadistic parents find all sorts of reasons to condemn their growing children; however, it is the rare parent who would admit that there are reasons to condemn their children because this is what the parent did to the child in the first place.

- An inner response to inappropriately high self-expectations that originate in the impossible-to-achieve dictates of one's own overly demanding ego ideal/conscience. A person with this problem often goes through life assessing his/her achievements not according to who the he/she truly is/can potentially be but according to the "someone else I might and ought to be." So this person routinely sees him/herself as a failure and feels and acts as if he/she has actually failed, then treats him or herself shabbily for being undeserving of most everything.
- Anger at others kept inside and turned around to become self-hatred, with anger introjected to become guilt and shame if only about feeling angry and kept inside due to the fear of losing someone if the anger should be openly expressed. Conversely, such people's complaints about themselves turn out to be complaints about others so that the sadomasochistic cry "I am worthless" often means "you did not act worthy of me," or the sadomasochistic plaint "I don't have what it takes" often amounts to "clearly that's why you don't give me what I want."
- Personality problems. Low self-esteem often originates in a sadomasochistic excessive empathy for and excessive altruism toward others, that overly sacrificial kindness that so easily turns to rage at oneself for not being properly directed or implemented and/or reciprocated, and the sadomasochist comes to feel that he or she is a big sucker who has once again allowed him or herself to have been taken in by others who are using the sadomasochist.
- A fear of success accompanied by suffering from survivor guilt. This plagues them should they succeed in any area where a loved one, or even a hated rival, has failed. Such individuals choose to lead their lives uncompetitively out of fear. They become overly giving, excessively self-sacrificial individuals paralyzed by the zero-sum belief that should they win something, someone else will as a consequence lose that same thing/lose it all and perish. Such men and women are often, to their own detriment, willing to take the bullet meant for their buddy.
- The belief that if they don't get what they want it means not that they aren't being given something for any one of a number of reasons but that they aren't being sufficiently loved.

- Being victimized by a psychosis/psychotic people. Who knew that, as one person told me, all the criticism of me that was coming her way came from all the frogs sitting on mushrooms and the tutelary's being indiscreet croaking to tell my critics that this person was no good and that this represented the unvarying truth. And who knew that my editor-to-be got mad at me because I sat in an empty chair that she had reserved for her dead husband's coming around to visit.
- Getting depressed due to their hypersensitivity, which often involves a special sensitivity to threats to their status and so their self-esteem as well as to the potentials for deprivation/rejection/control and castration (phallic) that they see everywhere and in everyone as a threat to their position in life.
- They themselves being unusually angry people who have a tendency to be as critical of others as they are of themselves. Excessive anger is bottled up, kept inside or turned inwardly, and taken out on the self in the form of self-critical thinking that leads to the self-criticism that proceeds and is responsible for the fall in self-esteem ("since I hate myself it means that I am no good"). The next step here is a temper tantrum where the anger ball bursts and they attack others, generally personally.

Suicidality and Sadomasochism

Suicidality and low self-esteem are often related. Here are some manifestations of suicidality in the sadomasochist:

- Taking inadequate care of one's physical health;
- Developing occupational block;
- Developing a severe form of workaholism;
- Becoming reckless, often associated with hypomanic hyperactivity;
- Developing substance abuse/addiction;
- Developing a success neurosis consisting of defeating oneself at every turn as well as defeating those who are trying to help by degrading their potential helpers' ability and reliability—refusing to cooperate with potential helpers as they question these others' motives and challenge their methods (a patient in her 90s kept falling because she wouldn't accept her daughter's advice to get rid of a throw rug she admired, since no matter how good the advice was it still came from her daughter who by the very nature of the relationship would have to be someone who showed judgment that was impaired compared to her own);

- Acting out an ultimate form of self-hatred and hatred of another, representing the duality that is part of sadomasochism whereby a single act is a compromise between two or more drives, in this case the living out of a combination of rage and guilt in one compound maneuver, such as cutting one's arms;
- An ultimate but misguided gift to someone one loves (a suicide note that says "you are not at fault" and means it);
- As a note that says hatefulness indirectly (by giving that other person pain and making him or her feel potentially responsible), as a manipulative sadomasochistic attitude meant to hurt and get back at someone (e.g., "she will miss me when I'm gone" or "my therapist will suffer when my family sues him for not preventing me from killing myself") or as an indirect act of giving pain via a pseudo apology ("I'm sorry I had to do this to you, but I had no choice because of what you did to me");
- As a way to get unpleasantness over with, the typical sadomasochistic act geared to produce cloture at whatever the cost (e.g., prematurely making out one's will); and
- Part of anger restraint, holding it in and taking it out on oneself.

A clinical manifestation of sadomasochism is the fullness of this anger to the extent that anger becomes a primary feature in "all" sadomasochism and is often so prominent that anger excess virtually comes to equal what we might call primary sadomasochism. Though anger both at oneself and others is at the heart of sadomasochism, and indeed anger at oneself and others also constitutes the building blocks of most psychoses and neuroses, still most studies of psychological impairment, including studies of sadomasochism itself, don't emphasize the role that anger plays in the causation of mental illness in general or in sadomasochism in specific in its diverse psychological complexions. Even a casual hearing out of sadomasochistic people ranging from those also suffering from schizophrenia to those suffering from very mild psychological impairments of various sorts shows us that rage is the driving force behind many if not most symptoms of this and other psychological problems. Perhaps the issue of anger is sidestepped in the literature out of fear of insulting the participants (by seeming to be accusatory). Unfortunately, the denial of anger as a building block of mental illness leads away from specific treatment (e.g., pharmacotherapy aimed specifically at rage). This spares feelings but prevents the institution from having adequate remedies. Looking the other way in the case of anger may do more than merely relieve anxiety: it can also affect the lives of others as well as one's own life.

THERAPY

Anger is an acceptable emotion, and overlooking it leads to inadequate interventions, especially in the realm of that self-pity that is a chief manifestation of masochism, and the projection of defeatism outward to feel for others who don't need the soothing and are even insulted by it, leading to harshness toward those deemed "pitiable," which soon spreads to become bigotry and other forms of hatred. ("I feel sorry for you feeling like a big nobody" soon becomes "you are the big nobody that my feelings tell me you are.")

The unilateral nature of anger and hence angry behavior is a chief problem for sadomasochists. Thus, angry sadomasochists dump a perfectly good relationship without warning and when the desire to do so is prevailingly one-way. Often they do this as they accuse the recipient of the anger for overreacting, without recognizing who and what started the reaction and whether or not it is in fact a reaction that is appropriate or is actually an underreaction after all.

Simmering anger almost always builds to the point of spontaneous eruptions consisting of saying and doing things that would otherwise be withheld and even entirely forgone and forgotten. (This is typically the case of the sadomasochism associated with depression.) It is generally said that the underbelly of sadomasochism involves joy in hurting and being hurt, but as often it involves relief in being able to express one's anger at others and oneself to get it out of one's system, then to get away with it as justified for legitimate psychological reasons. From hence comes a great deal of the pleasure inherent in sadomasochistic activity. That is, being in and inflicting pain is not the only or even the primary goal of sadomasochism; pleasurable discharge/release of anger, both at oneself and at others, is another one, perhaps one that is of equal importance.

A way to reduce angry behavior toward oneself and others has to be found to mollify the hold of destructive anger on angry sadomasochists and their victims. In view of the fact that sadomasochism is in some ways the obverse of empathy and altruism, a healthy helpful if indirect way to deal with the anger problem would involve enhancing altruism and empathy: always asking oneself, "what is my nastiness doing to him or her?" Another good place to start would involve reducing the narcissism that is at the root of much hurtfulness to others, disturbing their peace. Narcissism is at the heart of anger because it involves not "what I do to you" but "what you do to me," and this often involves "crossing me" in some way or another.

Correcting perceptive distortions becomes the remedy, leading to one at least becoming less angry, and that alone can lead to a change in sadomasochistic relationships along the lines of improvement of the nature of and the behavior in one or both members of a dyad. Correcting perception is often best done after identifying sadomasochistic behavior, seeing what just went before it (i.e., triggered it), leading up to it even just in the nanoseconds before the angry discharge. For some sadomasochists this is incident-related, but for others only certain things make certain people mad, and the same thing doesn't bother everybody. In cases of sadomasochism, it is wise to know your customer and avoid doing things that are provocative (what makes him or her mad) for a given individual.

There are some people who see the best advice as unacceptable because they see it as control. Therefore, you might consider not giving them advice. This holds true especially in situations where you are being blamed or at least dumped on for something over which you have no control.

Sometimes sadomasochistic behavior is covalent diagnosis-related, in which case it is wise to recognize people who are, for example, borderline and passive-aggressive and be therapeutic in a way that helps them with their underlying diagnosis.

Or you can recognize that there is very little that can be done except possibly stay away. As Oldham and Morris say, "transfer" from a job or "move out" of the home.[4] I was just dumped by a borderline I liked very much, but I got upset over nothing because I recognized that it was coming and did so right from the beginning, because it was the nature of the beast to see that there was no way to avoid such an incident. Passive-aggressives can be managed to some extent incident by incident, but borderlines will be borderline, and all relationships with them are likely to be stormy though often temporary, as they emerge after merging, a process innate to the borderline problem and not likely to be capable of being influenced by anything one does or doesn't do or says or omits in regard to the patient with such a problem.

Looking at the problem from the other way around as a practical matter, all depressed men and women should be examined for sadomasochistic tendencies involving violence to themselves and others, and all men and women who are violent/sadomasochistic to themselves and others should be examined for depression (and thusly treated by getting at the underlying anger and having the patient modify this, and if it is not modifiable at least to avoid elaborating the depressive trends simultaneously going on).

In summary, many sadomasochistic men and women are especially angry people, with their anger both of the appropriate or provoked kind and of the inappropriate or overreactive kind. In any event, sadomasochists stifle their anger, keeping it in and changing it into less harmful thoughts and actions because they fear that if they get openly angry others will not like them, and as masochists they wish if not to be liked then at least to be tolerated by all even though they pick those they already know won't like them in the first place.

Persistent unresolved childhood developmental conflicts, as psychoanalysis tells us, remain active throughout life as reflected in and so to affect adult functionality and create logical-seeming distortions that according to Oldham and Morris result from the progression from "what I think" to "how I feel" and how that determines "how I act."[5] Hence, when one is attempting to manage sadomasochistic anger, therapeutic interventions that offer understanding—particularly when coupled with cognitive corrections—can lead to remedies that can be at least somewhat effective.

6

Sadomasochistic Groups

MAINLY-MASOCHISTIC GROUPS

Sadomasochism is a notable quality in many political groups of today. As far as the psychodynamics of these groups go, while many authors have gone into the reasons (causality of) *individual* sadomasochism and the role that sadomasochism plays in personal dysfunction, the literature is scanty as to the role that individual sadomasochism plays in creating *social* sadomasochistic dysfunction (e.g., how and why groups of individuals seemingly with like minds are formed and how even the whole of the culture these individuals constitute seems bent on destroying themselves and others en masse even when alternative approaches to problem solving in specific difficult situations are readily available, though they are only so perhaps with some degree of difficulty).

Studying the makeup of sadomasochistic groups ultimately involves de-emphasizing the search for singular neurotic pleasure as it exists in the everyday lives, social or not, of the individuals in the group and studying why group phenomena supervene as a whole over individual motivation.

Sometimes sadomasochistic behaviors or other signs of mental illness are surprisingly absent in some groups. These "exceptional" groups often form around cultural factors, especially in societies where inherently protest is frowned upon such as the military, some bureaucracies, and some countries/parts of the world. Similar temperament, upbringing, native talent, and intelligence are factors in such a group's formation and functioning. The philosophy of the group is not necessarily a product of the group's shared psychopathology. Sometimes it is in particular the product of a pure search for power that may only be related distantly, if at all, to psychological illness. And the search for power is not necessarily the product of group psychology consisting of attempting to resolve individual conflict and so relieve anxiety on a widespread basis. The pursuit of the rewards of status and power may be enough to constitute the main factor involved—and be sustaining. Perhaps the Nazis were as a group as ambitious as they were paranoid. Power tempts and enables the individuals who hold it to carelessly blur the difference between right and wrong and to do so for political more than emotional reasons, each individual calling upon his or her version of right and wrong, hurting society but not necessarily doing so in order to reduce some anxiety of theirs and instead perhaps to fulfill their individual (possible biological) need for supremacy.

When groups (cultures) are formed around the principle that ego ideals can be shared, conflict characterized by hate may not be so much the core value of the culture and exclusion rather than inclusion not so much its core principle. There are, in other words, some groups formed through positive individual affiliation, the core of the group starting off by acting like a magnet that brings likes together, with others creating like out of unlike starting with a minor sense of shared love that the group first embraces and then enhances.

Groups may be masochistic or sadistic. As for the psychology of each group, masochistic and sadistic groups share one thing: a common philosophy.[1] Broadly speaking, the first, the masochistic group, has charitable features, and the second, the sadistic group, being in general a hate group, is one often based in hard attacks on others, often those others' race and religion.

Going into the psychodynamics of the different groups helps explain struggles involving class, race, gender relations, and alienation in this and many other countries.

Masochistic groups self-defeat to the extent that as a collective they are made up of individuals who have in common that they act sacrificially toward themselves. In contrast, sadistic groups as a collective have in common that they act sadistically, hatefully, toward other people by glomming together to be outwardly divisive—holding grudges, collecting injustices, devaluing all of others' accomplishments as insufficient, practicing haughty withdrawal, and writing rival groups off for little or no reason often based on assessments fraught with cognitive errors—and are also full of approval for themselves and full of recrimination for others and readily slip into other-directed anguish associated with powerhouse accusations of those around them, implying that others are to be devalued and responsible for all the bad that happens in the world, themselves refusing to take responsibility for any of this bad, instead insisting, in true paranoid fashion, that other people in their lives take responsibility for the misfortunes that are all around them, in the universe, and with delight inflicting narcissistic injuries on others of their sort.

In all events, everyone misses the opportunity for us all to work together to resolve differences, solve shared problems, and help people outside the groups that need the assistance that people inside the groups are, theoretically at least, in the best possible position to give.

So often the perverse inner world of groups drives them on to become hurtful to themselves and innocent others, holding them back from taking realistic actions they should take. They instead develop a group syndrome that resembles either a group depression (masochistic groups) or a group paranoia (sadistic groups) internalization and externalization of blameworthiness, respectively. And at times they make a good point or two and are instrumental for social change, but too often most of their ideas are platitudinous, and these goals are self-serving with a smile.

In short, masochistic and sadistic political groups may be composed of individuals less with like motivation and more with like mental illness, similarly troubled individuals who may be the product of a cadre of individuals with a similar personality or mental disorder.

Masochistic groups are activists who tend to let others and the world damage them without protest in situations where they should take control but instead, sheep-like, allow those bent on doing them damage or even taking their lives to get away with it.

Thus, minority groups involving what appears to be masochistic group psychology ask why so many Jews and Israelis delude themselves about the evil intentions of their enemies. (And if they retaliate it is usually weakly and with reluctance, as if the best they can do is in effect pull themselves up with their own bootstraps, allowing the groups' central, important ego ideals to be thwarted by other groups with conflicting hostile ego ideals.)

Unfortunately, great intragroup rivalries eventually occur, and groups generally dissolve in a short period of time, blurring one ideology and replacing it with another. Currently, who is hurting whom is the central concern (ego ideal) of many political groupings, and their goal is divisiveness, creating suffering, and forcing others to get out of the picture. (In a more all too rare positive climate, shared joy can be the goal, and divisiveness can be impermissible. This is not a prominent feature of today's culture.)

Motivating forces in determining the nature (complexion) of a given social group are always present, centered around hatred and not always clearly discernible as masochistic versus sadistic (depression versus paranoia). Characteristic at least of the more vicious groups are the following:

- They see the mote in their neighbor's eye and fail to see anything else in the structure of their surroundings except that which they chose to see and go on to elaborate; they get agitated easily over little things, especially those representing personal and/or social hatreds.
- They create adversarial situations where none are allowed to escape the hatred and be seen as innocent, or rational, as they manifest personal and/or social antipathies that come, however, mostly from within but are attributed to those on the outside.
- They view others from the perspective of how they view themselves—from within projected outward—so that when they call others racist they are in reality harnessing and trying to deny their own bigotry and attributing it to others. "I hate him" soon becomes "he hates me, and I am afraid of him," which can even become "he is hurtful to me."
- They decide whom they like and whom they don't like and reserve all their blame for the latter.
- Hypocrisy rules so that they get away with the homophobic remarks (referring to someone's aide as a butt-boy) they make without consequences while condemning others who make similar or the same negative evaluations, even getting them fired for being bigoted and in like manner.
- They feel persecuted by one person in another group or by the whole other group, and they believe that they are right and everybody else is wrong. Black and white are the only two colors they see, stop and go the only positions they can take.
- You can't talk them out of their distortions; trying to do so only makes matters worse as they dig in.
- They demand others agree with them or die; they show a propensity for making death threats of a potentially real homicidal and suicidal nature.
- They see and hear things that aren't there (e.g., the U.S. president landing on their terrace in his private helicopter three times in a month).
- The groups they form are only formed with those of a like mind at least in the beginning; soon afterward, however, internecine struggles disturbing the homogeneity occur, and splinter groups form.
- They see universal plots to destroy the world everywhere; nothing short of catastrophe interests them.

- They themselves can as a group have homicidal (murderous) and sometimes suicidal (self-destructive) tendencies.
- They are secretly attracted to those they condemn, though they say they want to be as unlike them as possible; that's why they are so preoccupied with the philosophies of their enemies, along the lines of it takes one to hate one. Homophobic groups often contain a number of latent homosexuals.
- They condemn people for not belonging (e.g., immigrants), distinguishing those who don't resemble themselves from those like themselves—those who do belong. Entrance requirements are stiff and remarkably similar for all without much latitude/variance permitted.
- Humans by nature desire adversaries; this is one function that groups fulfill.
- A shoulder to cry on is provided and is pivotal.
- The group offers companionship. Social individuals enjoy getting together. Social functions (e.g., dinner parties) are facilitated, and sometimes these are the major if not the only motivation of the group; positive feedback/congratulations are in order for like thinking. As my boss once told me, in my social group we all think the same and alike, and therefore there is no divisiveness, so we don't argue (for once).
- Out-groups are identified and "properly maltreated"; that is, they get what they deserve for thinking in a presumably aberrant way; the individuals in any one rival group are kept in check very effectively by outside group pressures.
- One sadistically maintains group adhesion by not condoning individuality.
- Ideas are replaced by rallying cries, generally repeated with little deviancy/development until they affect reality and enforce the same ideas. Development is frowned upon and treated as intragroup insurrection.
- Congratulations seem in order for intragroup-like thinking; personal criticism is avoided simply by remaining silent when one has individual ideas that prove the exception to the group's ruling philosophy. Creativity is dangerous; original achievements can only be accomplished by those who form adversarial relationships with other group members, leading to exclusion from the group.
- Loss of approval of one's peers is a powerful controlling deterrent, one that creates group adhesion; the group's basic idée fixe is enhanced through strength in numbers and supportive feedback, the nature of which does not deviate from some accepted predetermined norm.
- Attempts are more successful in changing so-called deviant society if one considers the power of the group as compared to the power of the

individual, which is relatively tiny. Characteristic is magnification in group formation, where molehills become mountains as minor issues get inflated to become major players, leading to attributing to others angry discomforting thoughts about oneself so that these thoughts are believed to be coming from others—and specifically those others who in their responses are in fact not just somewhat off the mark but are (considered to be) blamers. Here minutiae are inflated to assume gigantic proportions as some trivial matter takes over and runs the whole show, leading to omniscience whereby a sadomasochist rules about everything and yields to nothing, and the rules of the game involving having every potential discussion turns into an actual battle, and every major battle turns into an outright war soon to become manifest as a derangement syndrome.

- Funding is easier especially if the in-group is initially formed with funding in mind and its philosophy is honestly admitted as being directed to obtaining cash.
- Empathy is enhanced and involves understanding how another person feels; altruism involves putting this understanding into action. A shortage of both is generally found inside the group especially in relationship to outsiders. Sadism is enhanced toward the out-group.
- Contrasts are highlighted as generalizations, it being easier to identify and highlight aberrant thinking if it is multiple rather than singular in changing so-called deviant society and if one considers the power of the group as compared to the power of the individual.
- Ideational struggles are less meaningful for themselves than they are vehicles for hurtfulness of other human beings.
- Protest is of course characteristic of and natural to the sadomasochistic group. As with psychopaths who set out to get something for nothing, only to wind up punished (e.g., in prison) for their sneaky advantage-taking actions, sadomasochistic sadistic protest groups set out to destroy others (sadism), only to wind up hurting themselves (masochism) when the plot afoot, as eventually does happen, turns sour and things go against them.

Advocates

Politically oriented individuals are often passionate advocates, and it often seems to boil down to advocating for the poor (on the Left) against those who are lazy and shiftless and won't work but just expect handouts from the rich.

Masochism from the political Left, often liberal, may manifest savior complexes. These consist of sadistically shaming others for being inadequately altruistic and insufficiently empathic, at times exclusive and repetitive attacks geared to embarrass those who purportedly don't care enough for others who are suffering too, demands they suffer themselves in order to take care of those in need, willingly themselves sacrificing their own pound of flesh and giving it to those in need of it even though, or especially because, their altruism involved/commanded sadomasochistic self-sacrifice, so they are in a way not being at all altruistic unto themselves.

In some segments of our society in our occupational, political, interpersonal, and other socioeconomic venues, aggressiveness seems to be the norm. But as an example, in social groups devoted to protest, what looks initially to be purely sadistic may, as previously discussed, in fact be masochistic, with masochism manifest from the start by the recognition of the inevitably of being punished for one's advocacy (e.g., carted off to jail by the police), and sadism is often reflected from the start in others' sadistic permissiveness involved in refusing to punish an individual for his or her clearly manifest indiscretions, encouraging by not discouraging them, just to make a hurtful point.

A neighbor says, "I am so glad that I was the one chosen to be mugged. Yes, I was seriously hurt, and can never work again, but yes, too, I can handle that better than someone who is more ill-equipped to handling being laid up forever than I am. I have the psychological will and strength to integrate being disabled in my life, the psychic wherewithal to tolerate knowing that I will be paralyzed in my legs as long as I live due to the attack, and the financial resources to survive being out of work perhaps forever, or at least having to look for another job—one that I know I will be able to find, although I am not necessarily in high demand in any marketplace that I am currently aware of."

A mother lode of masochistic social protest runs through most forms of social activism, characteristically but not exclusively coming from the Left in the guise of some forms of activism relying heavily on this form of expression rationally justified as innocent, since it is philosophically and socially honest and useful in implementing a cause. Aside from its superficially innocent and socially unimpeachable quality, its sadomasochistic elements can stand out in the hurt and inconvenience it confers upon others and the ultimate self-destruction it confers on the self, sometimes many years later when the individual's self-sacrificial tendencies are recognized in hindsight and the individual holds him or herself accountable exclusively for the early effects of his or her self-defeating personality.

A masochistic society is based on the shared will to self-sacrifice and give to others (e.g., some marches). (Such societies do not survive when there are too many sadistic societies waiting to destroy them in order to purvey their own philosophy and fill their coffers with the money from their own people.) A society made up of individuals who consider empathy for others the first and only important thing may not be able to survive/cannot survive the inevitable self-destruction of self-sacrifice that so often to be satisfactory requires more than a large dollop/measure of self-abnegation as the shared ego ideal. (The ego ideal represents preference, and there is no accounting for taste.)

Attempts to overthrow the establishment are central to the group philosophy. Groups remain homogenous only when there is an alpha individual who leads the group, ideologically holding it together.

Self-blame followed by self-sacrifice turns into sadism when hatred is directed outward to create a disruptive social grouping where the main goal seems to be to make trouble, so that within a given philosophy that which is destructive is avowed to be constructive. Affixing blame and disfiguring those who are trying their best are the rallying cries. "Hate the leader" rarely becomes "Help the leader."

The group is being altruistic saying it is doing its work solely to help others with no serious concern for its own benefit. They seem masochistic in the sense that they tolerate their own adversity for someone else's good; careful exploration, however, reveals that self-interest is sometimes in their heart even though they profess that what they are doing and others are experiencing is for some greater social good, for example, the good of one's country. What happens to the funds they collect is sometimes another matter.

Is there any such thing as true altruism? There are some formal charitable groups that aren't beset by an underlying sadomasochistic motivation that is really the avowed purpose of the group, and that would include the many charitable groups whose avowedly admirable and avowed purpose is to help a specific person or a certain group of people, for example, those without enough to eat who suffer in the mountains from ringworm. There are no hidden motivations here, because the group members could just as likely rally around another cause as long as it is one of giving to others for some reason; in other words, an honest general nonspecific "giving" ideation motivates them, and its specific contextual setting almost doesn't matter. What matters is that sadomasochistic passion needs an outlet that, generally speaking, can shift from noble to noble cause and needs to be discharged as if it is a motivation that is primary in search of a raison d'être.

MAINLY-SADISTIC GROUPS

Politically speaking, a crude analogy is that right-thinking politics are more sadistic than left-thinking politics, which are more masochistic.

Sadistic groups are from the Right; if not overt/active in their negative intentions, they are subtly hurtful nevertheless. They say it is just another form of sadomasochism to simply wink (without condemning) at obvious need as self-induced. We hear that "the problem is that you refuse to work for a living," as if those who are hungry are in fact starving themselves.

A woman, a sadistic antifeminist, demanded being independent herself but held women who worked for her to a different standard, one destructive of their own personal strength and independence as people and as women. It was the standard that when she was an adolescent she held her own mother to. It was the housewife standard, the one that says that "Real women stay at home and cook and clean." She claimed she favored feminism, but her interest in being a liberationist only applied to her and, as a reaction formation, was a way to deal with her (poorly self-perceived) guilt about wanting women subservient. Ultimately her true colors showed in the form of her developing a sadomasochistic occupational inhibition, a typist's cramp that represented her own admitted masochistic "declaration of dependence"; that is, it was a way for her to "put down the pen and take up the broom."

Control and dominance are some of the preferred techniques of sadomasochism from the Right. Racist doctors in a medical clinic made a non-white nurse feel defective for being black by disagreeably correcting everything she said, to the point that she went home angry and depressed every night. When the nurse pointed out that an interviewee was beginning to cry, they corrected that to "no, she wasn't beginning to cry, she was 'beginning to tear.'" One prided himself on correcting her when she seemingly failed to adequately distinguish objective from goal, guarantee from warrantee, and opera from operetta and when she unforgivingly referred to Amtrak's Auto Train as the "car train."

A doctor in a medical group once asked this nurse, whose training and experience were considerable, for her diagnosis of a patient. When she gave it to him, he retorted, "What? You must be crazy?" The nurse naturally replied, "If you think I am crazy why did you ask me for my diagnosis in the first place?" The doctor then replied, "Because I didn't know until you gave this diagnosis to me how bad you were at diagnosing and how paranoid you got when people who are just trying to start a discussion with you even hinted that they disagreed, if only in minor ways, with what you thought and had to say."

Some groups on the Right are formed specifically to be sadistic toward specific others. A functional society needs to discourage such social Visigoths lest it will inevitably allow itself to be destroyed from without if not from within. These sadistic groups get where they want to go by being hurtful, perhaps by weakening or destroying rival groups, though the warlike core of their society maintains a semblance of peace and rationality to the outside observer. As with some forms of sadomasochism, the goals of some groups are illusory in terms of practicality. Just recently a number of students walked out of school and marched for school safety based on passing new laws for gun control. The motivation is admirable. The method is if only by default acceptable. But the results were negligible. The students were confounding effort with effect, as did those who marched for conquering cancer without asking for contributions. Walking hard doesn't halt metastatic activity, unfortunately. Most helpful is a certain amount of money being raised and put to practical use. Unless one believes in magic, other than that, the intense effort made in one area cannot be transferred to have an intensely positive effect in another. In too many cases, the sadistic feelings directed toward guns and those who make the guns and the gun control laws will have little to no deterrent effect on the outcome, which ostensibly among other things is to prevent school shootings. To have a maximal effect, the nonsadomasochistic fantasy must be directed as precisely as possible to the reality so that with "marches on poverty" producing income is a viable goal as it would be against any other social enemy where real points for one's actions beyond perhaps the publicity involved can be the most effective antidote sought. Perhaps it might be better to use the time to work at something remunerative and earn some money and give it to experimenters in a position to make great discoveries. Otherwise, this is suffering for a cause but not for a real result.

MASOCHISM IN WOMEN

The distortive picture of femininity and what it means to be a woman spills over into descriptions of masochism in women as a group.

Many studies have noted that women's and men's sadomasochism are clinically different.

For example, in regard to somatic symptoms such as anorexia and overeating and weight loss and gain, men who are masochistic tend to present their masochism as characterized by more somatic symptoms than women, for those latter ones are the symptoms for which, as Cochran and Rabinowitz note, it is "more acceptable for a man to suffer overtly because somatization functions as a defense against taking personal responsibility for life's predicaments" and because somatization is a way to avoid internal self-blame. And as for sadism, some observers would agree that the vast majority of perpetrators of violence are men.

On the other hand, Cochran and Rabinowitz note that some of the most frequently reported symptoms such as dysphoria, death thoughts, changes in appetite and sleep, fatigue, and difficulties with concentration—do not differ significantly across genders. Also according to Cochran and Rabinowitz, the frequency of occurrence of the first overt episode of clinically manifest sadomasochistic behavior might be clinically different in men and women, but "once sadomasochism-depression has developed, the nature of the disorder, except for a very few characteristics, does not differ at all."[2]

I have also noticed a different quality of the feel to men's sadomasochism portrait as compared to women's, one that to some extent represents the different presentation between the sexes based on the causal differences of sadomasochism between the genders. The woman, seemingly stunned by *loss,* has an abandoned feel to her sadomasochism, giving it a "woe is me" kind of portrait, while the man, seemingly stunned by a failure to achieve some ambition of his, displays an inability to feel in control or avoid the feeling that he is being castrated by a sadistic woman with a "vagina dentata," thus exuding a feeling of loss of masculine pride, the belief that he has been wounded to the extent that to the observer this imparts a sense of abject defeat, often one inclusive of a sexual nature. Some sadomasochistic women can't help but make it a practice of reminding us of a poor abandoned orphan who has just lost her parents and can't get mad (except to blame herself) except to say "look at me and see how much I suffer," almost as a badge of pride and courage, while many sadomasochistic men remind us more of a crestfallen peacock or of a prideful gladiator who has just been vanquished in the last battle he will ever fight in his life.

Gender-specific *group* personality differences to some extent also account for some of the individual clinical disparities here. In my experience, groups of men are more likely to have a paranoid (fight) response than women, and so in their sadomasochistic behavior men tend to be more irritable and violent to others, while women, being more all-suffering than men, are more likely to have a flight response. It is a stereotype, however, that men complain while women cry.

Some women think that honest expression of their woman's sexuality threatens the attainment of a desired love bond with a man (e.g., most men suffer from a virginity complex); therefore, women tend to underreport their true desires both of a moral and physical nature. Men are often sadistic to women who are perceived to have basic sexual drives, so women hide these in order to maintain the respect and hence the love of a man.

Finally, according to Deutsch, Horney contends that Deutsch regards feminine masochism as "an elemental power in feminine mental life and thus according to her view what woman ultimately wants in intercourse is to be raped and violated; what she wants in mental life is to be humiliated."[3]

REMEDY

As Oldham and Morris say regarding therapy, if you "find you cannot extricate yourself emotionally from a relationship with a sadistic [group], ask yourself whether you may have an unconscious need to suffer."[4]

Gone from this list is the mea culpa that might be the start of a useful discussion about what is wrong and what can be done about it, their failure to apologize for anything being one of their most prominent and most self-destructive traits. In other words, group insight is absent; we never hear "let's sit down and take a look at ourselves," only "lets stand up and fight against the enemies that surround us."

Groups, masochistic and sadistic, are dangerous because group power generally surpasses individual influence. Group demands, such as those focused on improving the environment, generally carry more weight than individuals who make pleas to grow vegetables in sanitary conditions, and retaliation for frustration can be cumulatively more swift, intense, and hurtful than anything most people can muster on a one-by-one basis.

IN SUMMARY

Here in summary are some ways the presentations of sadomasochistic anger manifest themselves as group phenomenon and make sadomasochists look as paranoid as they do sadomasochistic:

- They see the look in their neighbor's eye, and only that, and feel angered and seek revenge.
- They create adversarial situations out of situations when neutrality or cooperativeness in fact originally exists.
- They evaluate others as themselves projected from within onto others (e.g., they blame a spouse for the very infidelity that infests their own hidden wishes, which constitutes projective identification).
- They are full of hatred even toward those who are innocent as they come to feel persecuted by one person or a group of people.
- Their angry imaginations are vivid, they believe that they are right and everybody else is wrong, and they find arguments to the contrary to be unconvincing so that one cannot talk them out of their distortions.
- They demand that others agree with them—or else.
- They form groups of those with a like mind and extrude others (e.g., they only watch the television news shows where the content parallels how they think).
- They have personal and/or social hatreds, a cadre of people who become either their favorites or their bêtes noires.
- They see universal plots to destroy the world as being motivated by groups that are acting far less than innocently, though they just may be practicing their religion.

- They have homicidal tendencies that are sometimes but not always unconscious.
- They get agitated in situations where they should remain calm.
- They get depressed in situations where they reasonably ought to get angry. Some depressives are angry people who take their anger out on themselves (in the form of masochism) and express it at others (in the form of sadism).
- Sadomasochists who let their anger go a little often reach the point where their anger can't be stopped in time to rescue a relationship. (Therefore, sadomasochists at such junctures should be instructed to say less and instead work through in their mind what makes them feel so threatened in a given situation and do so before they say anything at all that can have permanent harmful effects on a relationship.) They should not feel as if they have to talk about what makes them feel the way they do, which could possibly lead to escalating anger that is especially dangerous for some sadomasochists with certain highly destructive propensities. It is true of most sadomasochists that if they let themselves feel a little angry they will let loose and become emotionally flooded, because all of their anger will emerge on the coattails of a little of their anger and flow outwardly until the ball of built-up anger bursts. Their anger after building will soak them through emotionally, resulting in their taking their anger out on all available objects, themselves in a masochistic fashion (which is anger transformed by being turned around on the self) or in a sadomasochistic fashion (which is anger transformed into plotted hatred of a specific nature directed to a specific other person or situation).
- They are secretly attracted to those they condemn and want to be like them (e.g., the rich people they envy or the poor people whom they condemn for being lazy).
- They condemn people for not being like them (e.g., immigrants). They have a propensity for writing poison-pen letters, even making death threats and otherwise expressing homicidal and suicidal fantasies.
- In the arena of expressing anger indirectly, sadomasochists overlap with passive-aggressives when they hold in their anger, when it might be a good thing or one would expect them to express it. They hold back their anger due to confusion about the appropriateness of feeling the anger and the belief that there are high costs to angry responses. The more passive-aggressive masochistic individuals believe that feeling and getting openly angry is at odds with a self-image that they wish to present

and maintain as good, which they equate with being all-suffering, so they routinely proclaim how anger in public goes against the grain of their personal preference and individual philosophy. Sadists justify their anger as having been provoked, thereby sparing their self-image as being of an evil nature.

PART 2

Causation

7

Causal Classification

An Overview of Various Pathways of Development

Sadomasochism is a complex phenomenon generally consisting of the later effects (residua) of many early developmental pathways occurring simultaneously or sequentially, making it difficult to impossible to be certain of causation both in all cases and in any specific instance. Therefore, one must not oversimplify when discussing the causation of a specific individual instance of sadomasochism. As the child passes through his or her maturational phases involving innate and provoked issues, such as those regarding Eros and Thanatos (the life and death instincts), inner forces take center stage, and these forces interact with external events to form the earliest outlines of the picture of the adult sadomasochist in the making. According to Fenichel, "Freud [said that] there are two qualities of the mind: a self-destructive one, the 'death instinct' (which can be turned toward the outside world and thus become a 'destructive instinct'), and an object-seeking quality, driving for higher units, the eros."[1]

Bekes, Perry, and Robertson note that lifelong beliefs and interpersonal attitudes are laid down when individuals are children. As they say, what is emphasized is painful early attachments, early injury of self-representation, identification with an abusing parent, and narcissistic injury. These are all core experiences in the early childhood of patients with masochism.[2] Most authors described early global psychodynamic conflicts, developmentally early motives and both action-level and neurotic defenses in masochism. As Ehrmann says, "If Freud's theory is correct, children who have experienced spankings or whippings will tend to be, or would tend to want to be a sadomasochist . . . but other social factors such as repression and knowledge of the social norm, allow . . . for sadomasochism to be better understood."[3] According to Grimwade, Schopenhauer says that the will to live accounts for the understanding of a form of primary sadomasochism, or pleasure, or acts of other-directed cruelty, our *Schadenfreude.*[4]

The first months/years of growing up can have irreversible negative effects on children, especially if they are being taught cruelty to themselves or others at the hands of those who should be teaching them how to love but instead seem to reserve their deepest interests and most intense feelings for establishing and catalyzing adversarial relationships of spite and resentment early in life, whose character shows then and persists later in life from early adolescence to adulthood. As a result, those in need who expect succor from others find only competitive/hostile interactions, where one is fighting and the fighting is a product of rejection, control, and competition with rivalries that are unnecessary because getting along is theoretically possible in most cases. How much sharper than a serpent's tooth are the sadomasochistic interactions many parents find themselves having with the ungrateful child and having them even when there is no snake anywhere to be found?

The sadomasochistic adult fully becomes that way due to specific interpersonal events that occur in the formative first years of the child's life, as the child, interacting with his or her parents, siblings, other family members, caretakers, and schoolmates, grows up to become a bully because there is nobody around, such as a nonsadomasochistic aunt, to tell him or her how to behave and to stop all the hostility, enforcing the message that the best relationships are often of the kind that are the most positive and especially as regards matters of dependency, control, and competition with others in the family, friends, and spouses. In addition to parents, siblings come into the picture in many ways and often along the lines of exemplifying and intensifying the core vindictiveness and spite of sadomasochism, and as an aspect of development this is generally overlooked.

Sadomasochistic relationships work two ways; this is not a one-way street. What the child contributes to the relationship with his or her parents is as important as what the adults contribute to the relationship with their children. Paradoxically, the child who loves too much is possibly as at risk for becoming a sadomasochist as is the child who hates inordinately.

CLASSIFICATION ACCORDING TO DIFFERENT DEVELOPMENTAL LEVELS (KERNBERG)

Kernberg emphasizes how sadomasochistic behavior in adulthood may be classified in a number of ways, each of which throws a different light of understanding on one or more aspects of the behavior we are attempting to identify, sort out, and comprehend—patterns of behavior we need to observe to be successful in our quest to bring order out of the chaos of this multifaceted problem of everyday life/symptoms of this emotional disorder and to successfully treat its more prominent and more dangerous manifestations.[5]

Kernberg emphasizes that sadomasochism is to be understood in relation to different developmental levels that are reached during ongoing childhood growth and development. Some of these (not as emphasized in the literature) are events that take center stage before and after a central period.

While the residua of early levels of development foreshadow specific adult sadomasochistic manifestations (symptoms), these manifestations do not, however, co-opt the entire personality so that a given individual is still left to function in nonsadomasochistic ways in important areas of his or her life. Throughout, we must always remember that the mere presence of a mental illness, even a severe personality disorder, doesn't necessarily disqualify an individual for functioning effectively in many of the venues of his or her private and public life. Bad sadomasochists often make good overall effective leaders.

CLASSIFICATION ACCORDING TO PRIMARY LEVELS OF MASOCHISTIC PATHOLOGY (KERNBERG)

Since every developmental stage contributes to the formation of sadomasochistic symptoms or character traits in the adult, we need to be clear about the special origins of sadomasochism in any given individual in order to know how and where to focus our diagnostic formulations and treatment planning in a given case.[6] Specific developmental occurrences contribute to/stamp the later (sadomasochistic) character so that we might have an oral sadomasochist who becomes angry and vengeful over issues of abandonment, an anal sadomasochist who is primarily invested in controlling another person in a dyadic relationship, or a phallic sadomasochist who is primarily concerned with and gets angry in relationship to matters of competition. The outcome to a great extent depends on the developmental level of the psychic apparatus during which significant, often traumatic, events occur and the degree to which aggression predominates over libidinal emotions/experiences.

Many individuals have later become sadomasochistic in essence due to having had negative (traumatic) experiences with primary caregivers from early childhood, especially experiences that lead to a negative response/an unempathic hatred toward the mother. According to analytic theory, several important defenses early on come into play vis-à-vis one's relationship with one's mother. The negative affect toward the mother is partially *repressed* and then is *turned into its opposite* (longing loving feelings toward the mother). Ambivalent feelings result; only then, later in life, is the negativity subsequently displaced outwardly to and relived in another relationship (e.g., one with a partner or in transference to the therapist in therapy).

Attachment (who I love) and self-esteem regulation issues (am I worthy?) are primarily affected, because they are among the most active in the first few years of life. Lifelong problems may thus be the result of the effect on relevant areas, causing particularly persistent problems with others due to experiencing difficulty with dependency, which may be atretic (e.g., undeveloped), or difficulty cooperating with others due to a pathological need by the ungrateful child to be the one on top in various struggles, the winner in various battles, with the final common pathway being a distortive self-view: "I am a bad person and as such someone who needs to be punished for my (presumed) evil motivations and misdeeds"—a child virtually inviting punishment by others for how he or she misbehaved and/or provoked and otherwise mistreated those who loved him or her. And on their parts, the parents in the history of too many children's development turn out to be competitive parents who almost reflexively try to convince the child that he or she is always wrong and the parents are the ones who are always wronged. It is important to recognize that oedipal conflicts work two ways: the child envies the parent and wants what he or she has, and the parent envies the child and wants what he or she still has.

Children with different parents and caretakers living in different parts of the world with different cultures manifest the residua of these different cultures later in life. Different societies take over a child's growth and development and rule in different ways, imprinting their special patterns upon the infant/child.

A major truth is that the first months/years at home are the ones that have the strongest irreversible effects on children, especially those who are being taught cruelty to themselves and others at the hands of those who should and sometimes even do love them. As the child interacts with his or her parents, siblings, other family members, caretakers, and schoolmates, he or she is affected by those who bully him and vice versa. But this doesn't mean that the child doesn't change after the first few years; life psychiatry theory says that the reverse is the case. Perhaps sex and aggression and in particular oedipal sexuality are most formatively meaningful early on, but later in life new and meaningful trauma also contribute to the final picture.

It is as possible to become a sadomasochist due to aggression and or erotic conflicts, and the tolerance and intolerance of one's Thanatos count for as much as that of one's Eros. Vindictiveness and spite are as important as, intertwined with, and all-consuming to the preoedipal and oedipal child as are the familiar and much-overemphasized problems associated with suckling, toilet training, and oedipal rivalry. The child's temperament counts too (i.e., what the child contributes is as important as what the parents contribute) so that the child who is remote and distant might be as much at risk for becoming a sadomasochist due to parental input as would be the child who hates inordinately and for little or no reason, affecting how the parents treat him or her. Some children are too self-protective; others are too paranoid, responding in warlike fashion or with remoteness to any attempt to understand/relate to them (e.g., asking them a simple question hoping for a revelatory answer).

CLASSIFICATION ACCORDING TO LIFE PHASES OF SADOMASOCHISM

The following statement applies to most or all of us: Throughout life, and often on a daily basis, we are placed in the impossible position of having to respond to the sadomasochism of others. As most psychiatrists agree, destructive acquiescence in the sadistic or masochistic possibilities inherent in certain situations from which escape is not feasible or desirable may occur with powerful people who claim or at least are supposed to be offering love. Here, sadomasochistic tendencies may emerge under significant constant or intermittent pressure of external events in a child who has previously shown no special tendencies in this direction and otherwise may not show signs of pathological accommodation until much later in life.

Even as children, we are tempted, if not forced, to endure or, in retaliation, inflict discomfort or pain on ourselves or others. In general, the greater the circumstantial pressures measured by duration as well as by intensity, the less likely are any resultant sadomasochistic manifestations to be pathologically significant. It would be a mistake, however, to assume that sadomasochistic manifestations are or will remain modest or temporary simply on the basis of their being circumstantially oriented (i.e., a response to the circumstances under which these tendencies first occur). They are being provoked now, but just because they are now being at first provoked doesn't mean that they will turn out to be transitional. Sometimes sadomasochism only becomes a way of life persisting into adulthood because the individual is traumatized later in life. In too many societies, aggressive behavior[7] is virtually the norm, and this seems to be truer and truer as the days go by and the functions of the superego in any given society are eroded in favor of social factors that themselves erode the culture by releasing id in all its primacy.

CLASSIFICATION ACCORDING TO TIMELINE (OF DEVELOPMENTAL LEVELS) (KERNBERG)

Various developmental events occur simultaneously in the growing child who is thus a cauldron of drives and incidences at any one (or more) period(s) of his or her childhood.[8]

What are the characteristics of a developmental level? There are several such levels, the most familiar classification being oral, anal, and phallic-genital.

Expectedly, a growing child will be differently receptive/motivated from time to time. One example of motivation at a given time is as follows: the masochistic character is being developed in order to deprive one's parents of pleasure and to take revenge on them, with the child learning to defy parental expectations by sabotaging his or her parents' plans for some or all of their offspring—and the child is doing so out of a spitefulness, which usually turns out to be at his or her own expense. The child's position is "You want me to be a doctor? Hence I have enrolled in school as a guitar player. I truly believe that you must do what you love. What loves you doesn't count. Don't you agree?"

A main issue is that during different developmentally infused levels the child grapples with different problems that he or she then resolves in a special, hence developmentally infused, manner, each characterized by specific developmentally determined healthy or pathological methods of operative interactions.

Not only do oral, anal, and phallic masochism or sadism variously prevail as the child grows older, but also at issue is the degree to which on each level aggressive realms of feeling/experience predominate over the libidinal as hate wins out over love or the other way around. The individual fixates upon special levels and then regresses to equally specific levels, so we see, even in the milder examples, forms of behavior derived from being abandoned, being controlled/in bondage, and having competitive interactions with almost everybody—important or unimportant, respectively, the masochist who broods that nobody loves him or the masochist who broods that she has no freedom to express herself perhaps because she is a woman not a man, so why not just give up and go into hiding, or the sadist whose life depends on forming like-minded group relationships that he or she submits to or reigns over so that others remain under his or her control, the latter the boss, as exemplified by the currently familiar helicopter mother.

Still, according to Glick and Meyers, Kernberg says that these are the elements and timing of the different phases and

> stresses the need for simultaneous analysis of (1) vicissitudes of libidinal and aggressive strivings, their relative balance and integration, with libido predominating in higher forms of masochism and aggression predominating [in] the more severe forms; (2) the role of superego development and the impact of failures of superego integration in the formation of masochism; (3) the level of ego integration—neurotic, borderline or psychotic—that influences the quality of internalized object relations; (4) the pathology of internalized relations; and (5) the extent to which normal or pathological narcissistic functions predominate.

Very early phases. Objectless unbridled aggression prevails; this is part of primary sadomasochism, a phenomenon conceptually equal to the concept of primary narcissism (i.e., it is "just there in the fundament").

The end of the first year. Next, secondary sadomasochism comes into play. The aggression becomes both self-directed aggression and secondary aggression/sadomasochism, which comes to involve objects.

Age 26 months. Children begin to experience sadomasochism as the sadism toward symbolized whole objects, which then becomes directed toward the self, the sufferer.

Prelatency period, 26 months to 6 years. The threatening nature of oedipal concerns calls regression into action as a defense, and with regression (from the phallic state) anal sadistic drive energies are recathected. That is, the individual unable to handle oedipal issues turns back to preoedipal ones to try handling those again, doing so especially because they represent a level of comfort. Who is fulfilled now becomes less important than who is being stubborn and resistant when others make demands.

Adolescence, 13 years of age to adulthood. Intensification of the anal sadistic drive organization that has been previously blunted by the defenses of the calm of latency occurs.

Masochistic braggadocio (tales of born pain, proudly told) prevail; this is a kind of tattoo mentality whereby the image of manliness, of courage, is generated by the display of pseudostrength (the scar on the cheek). The masochist's narcissism is served when he or she can present his or her pain as an experience without equal, the "no one suffers like I have suffered" stance. The relationship between pleasure and sadomasochism now becomes strengthened: sadomasochism itself = pleasure.

Adolescent sadomasochism appears to be in large measure a manifestation of the persistence in memory of parental introjects. These generally turn out to be *poisonous* introjects that in turn consist of the punishing parent confronting and disciplining the defenseless child. Duplicates of such a relationship may be sought in the outside world; this is a means to recapture and a measure of the process of recapturing the lost object. One loves/hates others in one's sadomasochism more or less exactly as one loves/hates one's mother. Therapeutically speaking, becoming less sadomasochistic means loving/hating one's mother less, one reason why it can be so hard to become less sadomasochistic even through the best therapy with a motherly therapist.[9]

CLASSIFICATION ACCORDING TO COMORBIDITY

As discussed throughout, although not necessarily as a classification according to Kernberg, this is a way of classifying sadomasochistic behavior emphasizing organization around familiar pathological entities, often their developmental ones. The commonality here is the self and other defeating behavior, in each case presenting in its own way in very personal different styles, each of which in turn makes us think first of one of our familiar syndromes besides and in addition to sadomasochism (e.g., the obstructionism of OCD) or the suspiciousness of paranoia (in each case the sadomasochism takes on a different form, such as avoidant or paranoid):

- Paranoia, where the sadomasochism is organized around (characterized by) vendettas against the self (often after doing life searches) and others (where reasons for being negative toward and condemning people as individuals or groups of individuals are of primary importance though based on misattributed misbehavior of self and others, often rationalized and frequently involving issues of hate in the form of bigotry, generally denied as a simple evaluation of reality with an accusation starting with "If this were true . . . thus," letting the accuser off the hook in case he or she is caught lying;
- Borderline states, where the sadomasochism is organized around phasic shifts from hatred of others to self-blame (and hence withdrawal from others) and back again (cycles of hateful hurting to loving merging then back again);
- Passive-aggression, where the sadomasochism is organized around keeping hateful interpersonal interactions indirect but subtly accusatory;
- Depression, where the sadomasochism is organized around whining by patients who believe they have both too little of some things (love) and too much of others (enmeshment), often accompanied by devouring others with one's own high-pressured give-to-me demands, alternating with ignoring others as a way to hurt them; and
- OCD, consisting of a series of compromise formations where the patients believe and become angry about little things, things that

> hardly count, turning these things into big matters that, though they are little, are the very matters that for this person seem to matter the most.

Because of comorbidity, the setting of the sadomasochism is often as central/crucial to understanding the process as the sadomasochistic behavior itself. Compare, for example, sadomasochism in depression and sadomasochism in mania, where whining is significant in the first and overreacting in an accusatory fashion is significant in the second. In differing settings, the complexion of sadomasochism varies according to judgment, insight, and affect, and we also see characteristically polar opposite behaviors that occur simultaneously or sequentially in the same person, as the same individual sometimes displays the hyperphagia of bulimia (where the sadomasochism is displayed via overeating), sometimes the hypophagia of anorexia nervosa (where the sadism is manifest in a refusal to eat when required/demanded one do so), and sometimes both (binging).

Comorbidity also affects prognosis. Thus, sadomasochists with obsessive-compulsive personality disorder in order to hurt their therapists tend to display a negative therapeutic reaction (masochistic triumph) where the patient responds to improving by feeling worse: the masochistic triumph displayed/marked by the little smile that says "See, nobody can help me" or the sadistic triumph that says "What good can a defective therapist like you do for me?" Patients with cyclothymic personality disordered–features often show their sadomasochism in a way characterized by affective bipolarity; thus, we see a denial of sadism where the patient kills with kindness, alternating with a denial of masochism where bad luck takes center stage as the explanation for what just happened, presented in the form of "I am not out to hurt myself, it's just that good things never seem to happen for me."

Narcissistic masochists put their parental introjects out there for all to see, showing off poisonous introjects to let everyone know how terribly their horrible parents behaved toward them. This also gives the child the opportunity to inflict pain on parents who are likely not as bad as the child thinks and says they are. The recovered memory era with its paranoid implications showed us how emotionally charged retrospective distortion can affect one's memory, turning a perfectly ordinary or even positive child-parent relationship into a scenario of terror that was never warranted, as the so-called real horrific events described never occurred. Courtroom distortions (e.g., false accusations of any number of things) are often engineered by the same sadomasochistic diathesis/primary driving force/process: the wish to hurt comes first, and the reasons for hurting and being hurt come later, seemingly to justify a conclusion ready to go and in search of facts to back up the fiction. Narcissism is such a central aspect of sadomasochism that many observers conflate it with the sadomasochistic disorder itself. This can happen when "my pain is presented as an experience without equal" (e.g., a "no one suffers like I have suffered" stance is assumed). In such cases, the relationship between pleasure and pain now becomes clear. In narcissism, sadomasochism has become a source of pride expressed toward others, a great accomplishment along the lines of "Can you top this?"

CLASSIFICATION ACCORDING TO THE PRESENCE AND NATURE OF COGNITIVE ERRORS

Learning about the belief systems of sadomasochistic patients suggests a cognitive approach not only to understanding but also to treating their sadomasochism in the hope that all persons involved will yield to reason, figuratively and literally.

Cognitive errors give the punishing parent the opportunity to confront and discipline a defenseless child while seeming to be doing the right, reasonable thing on the part of all concerned. Personal guilt invades the parent's judgment, but there is no getting away from the true motivation of the parent, which is also to make the child feel bad about something. Typically, a parent also withholds congratulations as if they are not in order, doing so even though the child has behaved admirably and earned kudos, but the parent figures out a seemingly good reason to complain that the child has been refractory and so deserves punishment, certainly not congratulations for having done his or her best. The nature of the child's misdeed is easily though faultily conceived as a derivative, to use an analogy, of the equivalent of "mentally touching yourself down there."

Sadomasochism is related to guilty thinking and so is profitably viewed as being in great measure the outcome of having guilty thoughts, with blame hovering in the background at all times.

The pain and suffering of sadomasochism are perceived to be punishment for forbidden unacceptable oedipal desires and preoedipally related libidinal desires and aggressions; often self-punishment is installed to mollify or avoid the perception of, or actual danger of, retaliation and hence the damage to the self via abandonment by loved ones. The sadistic superego needs to punish and the masochistic ego needs to be punished out of an excessive unconscious sense of guilt, with the pain being payment for past transgressions and permission ("money in the bank") for further transgressions.

Here is a sample of some specific cognitions representing guilty preoccupations that pertain in individuals who are sadomasochistic—guilt forces that lead both to self-destructive behavior and retaliation toward others who, as the individual sees it, made one feel guilty for behaving the way he or she did. The sadomasochist's hope/ideal of a partner in a dyad equals not getting away with anything but always being punished appropriately for one's transgressions, which are various and omnipresent.

One persuasive cognitive error that sadomasochists often make involves the erroneous belief that needing something and getting something must per se be associated with suffering; another is the erroneous belief that getting something for oneself is always at another's expense; a third is the erroneous belief that if a need is significant, then it is inappropriate just by that quality/definition (of being excessive) alone; and a fourth is the belief that excessive pain is conducive to good morality and even moral triumph. Sadomasochism thus takes the form of complaints, justified or not, involving different rationalizations for various personal and presumably unacceptable social attitudes and beliefs; thus, "You have no right to point out a beautiful new baby on the cover of a magazine because that only reminds me of how many sad children there are in this world" and "of how I just lost my only child."

To anticipate, here are some other commonly made cognitive errors, also discussed in Chapter 13:

- The erroneous (zero-sum) belief that hurting others is the necessary accompaniment of achievement so that the individual comes to believe that getting something for oneself per se as a consequence inevitably hurts others.
- The erroneous belief that needing something and getting something ought to be/are per se associated with suffering. Perhaps parents pass on the message that nothing comes easy in this life, for everything is a struggle. The children are repeatedly reminded that they owe their food and clothing, their home, to their parents' toil and sacrifice. The child is made to feel thankful for every little thing he or she got then and is to get now and in the future.
- The erroneous belief that one's needs, just because they are meaningful and significant, are thereby excessive or inappropriate. Any need, however legitimate, is seen as excessive (outlandish) just on the surface of it. A child's needs are always seen as excessive and deserving of punishment, for all children make excessive demands, and therefore all children come to worry that they have been unacceptably selfish.
- The erroneous belief that pain is conducive or even essential to physical and moral superiority. (Sadists seldom think of themselves as reaping the benefits of physical and moral superiority through inducing pain in others; they instead see themselves as acting in the interests of the victim. Sadists who believe otherwise are likely to be psychopathic.) This idea finds its highest expression in certain forms of philosophical

asceticism. It is also implicit in the doctrinal accompaniment to the philosophy of rigorous elite schools, especially those that use caning or its modern-day equivalent as a corrective. In these institutions, the do-or-die ideology, inseparable from the institutional purpose, tends to obscure the thin line between the acceptance of discomfort as an inescapable fact of life and its glorification as a builder of character. The hierarchical structure of these organizations gives everyone the opportunity (or the expectation of an opportunity) to give and receive beneficial punishment. Belonging in this category are some analysts who undergo a rigorous but overly long training psychoanalysis as a rite of passage, as it does in hazing; graduate school, where the degree not the experience is the thing; and various unpaid internships undertaken for the experience in situations where there is no discernible fixed relationship between learning and overdoing. Social "repairs" that are in fact socially destructive are often inspired by the belief that there is no gain without pain.

- The belief that imperfect = no good at all, producing the wish to punish certain people (e.g., political figures) for not doing a job flawlessly, even one that cannot be done perfectly; therefore, if a leader suffers from a narcissistic personality disorder, this means that he or she cannot function as a highly placed leader of man in *any* shape or form. The protective and creative aspects of narcissism are overlooked/ignored depending on motivation, and changing one's life due to rethinking one's positions is considered to be a flaw/sin.

Also of classificatory value and therefore of causal enlightenment is the degree to which childhood aggressivity predominates over childhood libidinal forces of attachment (e.g., the negative oral, anal, and phallic aggressive over the parallel-running loving drives). The matter of degree to which certain elements are seen as contributing to the entire picture helps mold the very temperament that is at the heart of the child's sadomasochistic attitudinal approach to life. The individual first fixates upon and then later regresses to a level that is proven comfortable for him or her. In the milder examples, we see such sadomasochistic behavior as snappishness over imagined rejection, favoring being a controlling person by the child who presumably also won't mind being the object of control, and a nastiness originating in a competitive interaction with friends and family. In its more severe forms suicide or mass murder to take revenge directly obtains. In one case, a mother wrote her three daughters to come visit her now because in several weeks she is going to go away, never to be found again, and gave no further explanation.

The complexion of the final outcome depends on combined factors: personal preference (choice), external input (parental and sibling provocation and response), and inherent personality makeup. To some extent, the picture of the final outcome is preordained as a stereotype. For example, an intense angry temperament in an individual who lives in a gun-toting society out West and feels defensive because of hostility on the part of a given parent or from his or her siblings and additionally possesses a strongly mesomorphic body type may be/is likely to be interpreted as being a Thanatos-positive sadomasochist compared to others with more ordinary, more positive behavioral Eros-type characteristics. But surprises do happen, and rare exotic outcomes do occur—and almost invariably elicit a measure of shock in the room. For example, "She is the last neighbor in the world I would expect to be so full of hate. That she would pick up a gun and shoot her whole family is inconceivable to me; why didn't she just pick up a pen and write to her congressperson?" Questions of motivation are routinely asked and, because observers are not looking for cognitive errors, rarely produce answers/material that constitutes a contribution to a proper enlightening reply. Cognitive errors are discussed in greater detail in Chapter 13.

8

Classification According to the Level of Psychiatric Illness

The Psychotic Spectrum

GENERAL ORGANIZATION ISSUES

Speaking psychodynamically, according to some psychoanalysts, sadomasochism can be classified according to certain aspects of psychopathology that prevail now based on the relighting of specific crucial pathological developmental/traumatic moments that occurred then; Kernberg emphasizes the roles played by the libido and aggressive instincts, the superego, and the presence of neurotic, borderline, or psychotic features and internalized object relationships.[1]

These are in turn characterized and influenced by the level of development of the child when formative insults (traumas) first occurred (e.g., those that occurred at a time when the child might have been the most vulnerable). One example would be abandonment during the critical first few months of life, clearly affecting internalized object relationships.

The degree of personality organization (e.g., borderline versus nonborderline) and integration of the various facets of maturity and immaturity of the psyche relative to each developmental level counts for a great deal. The following different types of personality organization are distinguished accordingly: psychotic personality organization, borderline personality organization (low and high level), neurotic personality organization (particularly considering the possibility of strong narcissistic personality trends), and a post-traumatic personality organization due to primary traumas. These different possibilities represent/are the different contexts in which sadomasochistic (relational) behavior occurs or emerges. Thus, we might have a sadomasochistic borderline individual or a sadomasochistic narcissistic individual. We might see oral aggression of an organized nature, oral aggression in a disorganized personality, or phallic aggression in an organized personality (along with seemingly correct but in fact false accusations/recovered memories of parental abuse) or in a disorganized personality. The following realms are to a great extent distinguishable.

PSYCHOTIC PERSONALITY ORGANIZATION

When sadomasochism occurs within/accompanied by a severe level of psychotic personality organization, it is probably best to classify the disorder according to the psychosis to which the sadomasochism belongs. (In their turn, all or almost all "psychotic" realms present with either masochistic features, sadistic features, or features of both, in the sense that any of these illness/patient types can hurt themselves, others, or both themselves and others.)

The picture of sadomasochism within a level of psychotic personality organization is marked by fixation upon and/regression to primitive behaviors that the child may originally have found to be adaptive but, when maintained in the adult, suggest a serious level of ongoing decompensation (e.g., severe temper tantrums of today resemble similar ones from yesterday). The sadomasochist finds these levels to be "useful" as fixation points to slip back to when the going gets rough in the here and now and there is present tension that can best be relieved if extremely self-destructive methods are used to, for example, distract one from what one is going through now (e.g., earnest self-mutilation such as bodily self-destruction as a way to express one's personal rage by cutting, anorexia, head banging, breath holding, and serious suicidal activity, all distractive mechanisms there for the patient to use when anxiety builds and tension becomes unbearable). These methods serve not only as a distraction mechanism but also as a discharge mechanism so that the sadomasochistic behaviors provide the individual with a mechanism of relief from what would otherwise be an unbearable buildup of anger and become the equivalent of a discharge of sexual tensions that have accumulated or might otherwise build up to the bursting point over time and explode, perhaps as a way to attack others for what is believed to have been parallel earlier assaults.

Certain "crazy" beliefs such as those about being surrounded by inhabitants of the spiritual world often have a psychotic sadomasochistic core, depending on what these spirits happen to be doing to one or another involved person at the time and the degree of preoccupation with their presence.

Many of these behaviors such as head banging and breath holding can be understood psychodynamically as a compromise formation between hurting oneself and smashing into others with homicidal intent.

The tight structural nature of some psychotic behaviors can sometimes reflect their thoughtful nature, which puts these on a higher level than diffuse polymorphous perverse behaviors that simply represent random discharge of a primitive sort, as exemplified by certain sadomasochistic sexual activities involving urine and feces (such as those that take the child back in time to when he or she was a toddler smearing feces to get back at the mother).

In conclusion, this picture of sadomasochism in a psychotic setting is marked by fixation upon and regression to primitive behaviors that the child may originally have found to be adaptive but when maintained in the adult suggest a serious level of decompensation such as chewing one's integument that resembles a baby's putting its foot in its mouth and keeping it there for purposes of biting into and destroying the toenails. The sadomasochist finds these behaviors to be useful as fixation points to slip back to when the going gets rough in the here and now, and reconstructive methods show us that there is tension that can effectively be relieved if extremely self-destructive methods are used to move on from the here-and-now tension by invoking the same sort of releases that worked in the past. To illustrate, compared to what an imprisoned child (e.g., one in a seclusion room in a psychiatric ward) is going through now, earnest self-mutilation with reversible bodily self-destruction can be a comparatively safe way to reduce/express one's personal horror about something specific, cutting can seem to let the rage pour out, and anorexia can represent hate-filled oppositionalism that takes the form of starving oneself to death no matter how hard a caretaker wants or demands that the behavior stop and the patient resort to other methods of expressing rage, methods other than the primitive irreversible self-hurtful behavior such as a hunger strike.

Milder versions of these behaviors of course occur, as each has its equivalent/representation in normal behavior, such as head banging = knuckle cracking.

Walking it back, many "psychotic" activities are either masochistic, sadistic, or both in the sense that one hurts oneself, others, or both oneself and others so severely that any diagnosis of lesser import than "sadomasochistic psychosis" would seem to be inadequate to describe the nature and severity of the problem.

BORDERLINE PERSONALITY DISORDER

In the merging-emerging borderline sadomasochistic patient, behaviors such as hostile engulfment of others (enmeshment) alternates with equally hostile avoidance and rejection of others. This characteristic behavior in the borderline world makes some borderlines look like the patient with severe avoidant personality disorder of the characteristic merging and emerging of "I love you, now go away, come back I love you" sort, the world where patients alternate between unpredictable extreme closeness and extreme distancing, which in its modified form can present as the world of daters never being able to meet a companion for themselves, at least one who lasts for very long (e.g., until a new connection is made, only to be soon followed by their ridding themselves of the person as rapidly as they can perhaps because they have met someone else who likes them better and whom they like better in the first place). This behavior is self-defeating; additionally, it is often hurtful to others who don't understand what literally and figuratively hit them, that is, why they were so rejected. In a recent case a close friendship shook on the grounds that the woman was seeing her entire body swell up from eating the probiotics I suggested and then developing an alcohol withdrawal syndrome that would keep her from socializing on my level. This characteristic borderline personality organization also reflects hypersexuality that is in fact less sexuality than a loveless capacity for that component of sexual enjoyment that is called but is a false face of love. (Within some gay male worlds borderline hypersexuality involves attending bookstores where the chief activity consists of looking through peepholes at the next patron's masturbation and masturbating themselves, ultimately leaving all unsatisfied.)

It is not hard to attribute a sadomasochistic component to most if not all individuals with this basic borderline personality structure. Common descriptive and causal elements exist, as do the symptoms that Oldham and Morris suggest all borderlines show: "fears of abandonment, interpersonal relationships marked by extremes of overvaluation and devaluation, identity disturbances so intense that these individuals don't know who they are and where they stand and what they stand for in an already confusing environment/world often resulting in an as-if kind of personality with seemingly make-believe existences, and having identity crises with relational and job impairment [sometimes] occurring at one and the same time."[2]

To carry the comparison with borderlines into a more detailed realm, Kernberg divides borderlines into those who are low level and those who are high level, as follows.

For example, an individual in his 40s, though he hasn't had a gig in over 3 years now, tells of how he is going to persist in his chosen career as drummer with a band because his mentor told him that it takes 7 years to establish yourself in the field and he is just getting started. This he doesn't say came to him as a general caution/warning in a statement in a conversation referring to problems in the musical field in general but instead says that it came as specific advice especially relevant to him, though he is a man with no special talents that would justify his waiting out the 7 years while he became famous, especially with few to no signs of progress in his professional career, one where nothing is happening to indicate that he is moving up the ranks to reach his goal. His is in fact a fantasy fueled almost exclusively in his imagination, because while it represents a good general rule for some (give it time and you will get where you want to go), it is inapplicable to him and his future because there are no signs of his going anywhere in his professional life at present, thus making the homily irrelevant to his particular individual situation. His represented a kind of concrete thinking: that to become a good professional drummer you just have to wait it out for 7 years, which he is dutifully doing. Only he was forgetting to tell himself/omitting the part that first you have to have talent and during this time period be going somewhere, if only on the slow track, not the one that says "dead end ahead."

Low-level borderlines. Low-level (severe) sadomasochistic borderlines not only self-mutilate, they also run a distinct danger of successful suicide as an accompaniment/manifestation/complication of their self-mutilations. Their impulsivity can take the seriously self-damaging forms of behavior that is less than fatal but extremely self-defeating, such as alternating relational merging and emerging that consists of behavior that is dangerously self-destructive to one's life, plus emotional instability that is a product of stable affective instability—for example, recurrently getting functionally depressed and often for not much reason at all, experiencing chronic feelings of emptiness ("it's as if I have nothing inside me") and feelings of severe boredom ("I have nothing to do when the sun goes down"), feeling intense anger that might be controlled only with difficulty and much medication, and experiencing stress-related paranoid or severe dissociative symptoms.

As is said of the little girl with the little curl right in the middle of her forehead, these individuals are good when they are very very good, but when they are bad they are horrid.[3] These can be very appealing individuals when they want to be, but when they no longer feel the need to control themselves or can no longer control themselves due to the buildup of internal pressure (generally feeling overwhelmed by closeness with someone or anger at something someone supposedly did to them), they devour those who would love them (oral-level sadomasochism), who as a consequence feel they are having their very souls ripped out of their bodies and feel abandoned, rejected, overwhelmed, and chewed up and spit out in tiny little pieces, when they have done nothing much wrong except tolerated and even loved others far too much and accepted them far too excessively and too trustingly and sometimes gotten involved with them too intensely, there being awful consequences that could not be foreseen and can no longer in the here and now be tolerated with any degree of comfort.

Some serious borderline sadomasochists must have ongoing support, because for them anything less than full support becomes full abandonment. Others who want to express themselves in disagreement of any sort become the enemy just as if they had hurt the borderline sadomasochist personally and even fatally by attempting to say what was on their own minds. For one borderline, such people were destroying his identity simply by the act of affirming their own. Feelings about being devoured, controlled, and beaten competitively get all mixed too. This is because for such sadomasochistic borderlines, another's self-expression equals completely defiling him, subjecting him to embarrassment and humiliation. Matters of devouring, control, and competition also got into it, as this borderline always needed to be in charge in a given situation; otherwise, he would strike out at a companion. The actual content of the communication coming from the specific mouth from whom it was arising was not important for such a person, for this person would react in the same way with everyone. He would bolt as soon as he felt trapped in any way, even just by another person's expressed opinion. When his dog bit someone, good advice to report the bite to the insurance company was given but discarded because "who are you to tell me how to run my life anyway?" Fearing being trapped by having an appointment he had to stick to, he would hire contractors and then cancel the dates as soon as they committed to him, doing so even when they were on their way to his house so that as a result they had nothing to do that day after having to go home because of the date change. He would also purchase up to five properties at a time and then cancel the contracts one after the other, regardless of what this did to the other people involved in the deals.

In a general way, in his demanding respect for himself he showed no respect for others. Thus, he would call a doctor friend and ask him to come up in the middle of the night, demanding immediate medical care for some nonurgent condition. He would regularly make suicidal attempts, then call as the doctor was out the door, telling the doctor that he was no longer thinking of taking his life. And finally, he would call me as a doctor, also in the middle of the night, to say that since he hadn't heard from his other doctor for a few hours he assumed that either something bad had happened to the doctor or the doctor had decided to no longer be his friend, and he soon afterward gave up on the relationship with the doctor/me because he couldn't live with/handle that level of ongoing possible personal rejection from people he himself loved too intensely and so too well, although no doctor deserved his admiration anyway because of the way that all doctors behaved toward him in the past and, as he observed, treated their other patients and even their own family.

Soon an argument broke out whenever someone tried to say "this is the way I see things." Clearly narcissism was getting into this level of sadomasochism too, since dyadic situations were routinely being converted into monadic ones, with his needs the only thing that mattered, center stage.

To date, I haven't heard from him for several months, and this though he moved into an apartment right down the hall from me in the same building I live in.

My constant reminder to myself is that no matter how much I liked him I couldn't get along with him for very long, which reflected the precise reactions that this level of sadomasochistic borderlines bestir in others: they ought to feel somehow guilty over the possibility that they have upset the other person by their own behavior, whereas in real life they only acknowledge/recognize that the other person has upset them and that the other person has no reason to be upset.

Sadomasochists on the lower level of borderline personality organization are clearly characterized by their inability to entertain the victim's plight in any of their calculations, so they sadomasochistically ignore the costs to others and to society of their own sadomasochism. Instead they expect others to simply absorb any loss, for their only consideration is whether or not they can do better by themselves by getting more from others whom they come in contact with the next time. Political fights that can be cruel and get personal often fall into this category, and seldom is forgiveness forthcoming, "let's shake hands" being considered to represent insufficient reparation for this level of hurtfulness.

Severe body image disturbances exist. A patient said that she felt and behaved like a shifting sand dune. "I am rotund, with long white hair. I wear a cape that obscures my features, and I glide when I walk. Sidling along as if I am a slow-moving apod, I seem to pass through closed doors and walls, disappearing as a grub worm might do, then unrolling, reappearing on the other side as if by magic." Any protests to this self-description were met by disbelief, putting the listener in an embarrassing position of not knowing how to listen or respond. Here the body image disturbance was a concrete way of saying that one is not in this world but instead is all rolled up into a ball to stay out of it, at least until one "gets to the other side."

High-level borderlines. High(er)-level (less severe) but still essentially borderline personality organization sadomasochistic individuals are marked by chaotic but often ongoing (and stably unstable) relationships characterized by a degree of predictable clinging, dependency as well as/often alternating with aggressive closeness of a demanding hugging nature, such as that to be found in extreme jealousy alternating with resolute resentful distancing, creating unstable though ongoing minimally sadomasochistic patterns of merging-emerging with insufficient clinical evidence of the presence/appearance of consolidating and organizing restraining superego functions (e.g., there is little regret and less apologizing due to guilt and hence very little evidence of unconscious remorse). This has to do with selfishness being a hallmark of their behavior. The man referred to above was asked, "Are you at all concerned about what you are doing to others, e.g., what you are doing to me?" In return, all I got was a blank stare indicating it would seem that he totally lacked comprehension as to what I was getting at and how both of us might be feeling/thinking under the circumstances.

To a great extent high-level borderline relationships are the product of restrained ambivalence so that the seemingly loving borderline individual soon comes to fire away in a manner that leads the other person to feel as if he or she has just been rejected, just the opposite of the way things should actually stand between two people in a dyad composed of individuals both of whom down deep actually love each other.

Too, in this level of dyadic situation one victim (or sometimes both of the victims) is characterized as indulging in persistent infantilism marked by shifting dependency and independence whereby it is characteristically hard to know what momentous-appearing trigger set off some equally momentous-appearing shift of affections, in each case both the trigger and the shift being of a trivial nature.

Many of these individuals seem to suffer from a disorder diathesis rather than a single disorder or even multiple disorders; that is, they seem prone to becoming now primarily sadomasochistic, now primarily paranoid, and now primarily depressed.

Milder forms of high-level self-defeating behavior are often present and characteristic—almost as if the pleasure principle rules are deliberately and purposefully suspended but not permanently relinquished, making is seem as if these individuals simply do not much care that they are ruining their lives and chances for a productive future by underweighing the importance of today's skirmishes as they possibly pertain to tomorrow and thus the potential future implications of current episodes in the here and now. Most serious is their progressive loss of objects so that friends disappear one by one, and when family members die off they are not replaced by former strangers or new close friends. Ultimately, few to no one wants them around, and they come to their senses, realizing that they have lost many loved ones at the same time that they have lost their appeal and so are having a hard time making new, even superficial, acquaintances. This factor alone is often enough to explain why these individuals are the ones who wind up in the nursing home while similar individuals, in many respects otherwise their equivalent, continue to enjoy life on the outside, there being one or many persons around who take up the cudgel for this latter group and fight to not put them away and to do what they can to keep them as functioning senior citizens still in the community.

Finally, characteristic of these high-level borderline patients is that in the middle of such semichaos they still may have the capacity to fall in love; establish deep and dependent, even clinging, relationships; and even evince a greater potential for stability of love relations/a leadership than more primitive borderlines have ever come close to having.

A high-level borderline was exemplified by how high-level borderlines still have relational problems, but they are those where all concerned get hurt due to irregularity, ambivalence, and the emergence of hatefulness in unpredictable ways, especially when things appear to be going well. This person could not go out of the house for reasons she could not explain. But otherwise she took care of her family/herself and even worked at being successfully artistic in terms of painting beautiful watercolors and making sculptural arrangements that went on display in high-level galleries and sold well. But her one and only child was homeschooled because the school bell frightened her; she had one brother who currently was awaiting the right time to apply for a scholarship to college, though he is now 60 years old and the right time still hasn't come; and she has a mother who dressed up including being overly made up to go to the supermarket so that the other ladies who went there too didn't think of her as an old unstylish person.

Unfortunately, the sadomasochistic elements of a personality like the one such borderlines possess are too often incompatible with fully achieved sensible and realistic long-term relational and occupational goals. Sadistic, they are always at risk from personal and sometimes legal retaliations, and masochistic, they often court personal danger in part through their self-indulgent and provocative behaviors, being prone, for example, to road rage, among one of the most damaging of the types of embroilments to which they are prone.

A high-level borderline suffered mainly from relationship problems that showed essentially in her relationship with the dogs she fostered. Her main work in life was fostering dogs that awaited adoption from her home to a forever home. Sometimes the wait was long, and of course the dogs became imprinted on her. Then when somebody who wanted the animal came to accept it for its forever home, she (deliberately) put the person through such paces that the adoption was in danger of failing, and most adoptions did fall through. She simply couldn't release the dog from the relationship and herself from the relationship with the dog, much as she couldn't release the relationships she had with some of her friends and lovers. This borderline might be called high level because she was being so masochistic to herself (keeping and loving an animal sometimes for long periods of time, an animal that was not and never would be her own) and not letting the dog go and being both sadistic to the dog, which wasn't getting the forever home it could have potentially had, and sadistic to the person who wanted to adopt the dog and by now had fallen in love with it but couldn't have it manifestly for some trivial reason/excuse or another, specifically advanced under the aegis of the rationalization that her purpose was to find the dog exactly the right home and not a place where the dog would be treated less than how well she was treating it (which she was not necessarily actually already doing in her own special way).

High-level borderlines often emerge from a working relationship after something goes wrong in their mentation, however trivial this something might be. I am now and then very close to a wealthy, attractive, charming, intelligent individual. I look forward to seeing her for many weeks before our essentially monthly dates. But when the time finally comes to meet, I find the relationship far too wearying and intense to be sustaining or sustainable. Here is an example of what can happen between us. Once I suggested that she serve me a small portion of a certain dish, Rock Cornish game hen, because even a small portion was "far too rich for me," whereupon she embarked on a half-hour explanation of how the dish couldn't be too rich because she didn't ever serve something that was rich because it had cream in it, and she knew that because she never used cream in anything. Still to this day she keeps reminding me that I was out of step because her recipe didn't contain any cream, and still to this day she keeps reminding me that in a general way I was wrong to so mistreat her because she had worked so hard to cook a beautiful meal, done nothing wrong, and certainly did nothing to mistreat me the way I implied she had. I didn't understand what exactly she was getting at until I realized that her communication to me was autistic because it contained a high degree of personalization, that is, my complaint about what she cooked, even though I didn't actually make the complaint in so many words, was a complaint—not about the food but about her, so that my concerns had nothing to do with what she said or did but were unacceptable simply because they were of the very nature of complaints, and only pure positive feedback was acceptable, with any complaint whatsoever of no merit simply because it wasn't in the nature of positive feedback. Adding to the chaos were other similar autistic complaints that were part of her overarching derangement syndromes, which consisted of tempests in teapots whereby she often broke down to the point that she wanted to squelch other people who simply challenged/disagreed with her in any way, even though at bottom she actually agreed with what they were saying and disagreed with herself.

Even high-level borderline individuals, narcissistic to the extreme, feel compelled to squelch other people who merely disagree with them in minor ways. They develop a retaliative derangement syndrome in the face of anything less than a full complement of positive feedback. Retaliation in the form of constant repeated personal attacks follow as comeuppances. Too sensitive to rejection for their own well-being, like many other high-level borderline sadomasochists, they seemingly are stuck in the oral sadistic phase and so must always have support, because they see anything less than full support as full rejection. Others who want to express themselves become the enemy for attempting to say what they think.

Another feature of such borderline individuals is that they set out to destroy others' identity as part of maintaining their own, affirming themselves by de-affirming others. When there is disagreement, matters of devouring, control, and competition get mixed in to the interaction, because for sadomasochistic borderlines even those on a high level, another's self-expression is a defiling of their identity, with maintaining their own identity as they exist in a confused world a high priority to keep them from becoming lost forever.

Sadomasochists on this high-level borderline level of personality organization are also generally characterized by a lack of altruism and empathy, as made clear by their inability to entertain their victim's plight, often one they have induced by their own behavior. An example is to be obtained from the two women who lived in adjacent townhouses. One's roof didn't drain properly because of the absence of a proper draining mechanism; that is, she herself had no downpour spout. She "solved" the problem by hooking up a mechanism whereby a pipe ran from her roof to the roof of the woman next door, then down into the street through that woman's drainpipe. Using her neighbor's space wasn't bad enough given the circumstances, for she could have easily installed a drainpipe of her own from her own roof directly to the ground below. But what she really wanted was a merger whereby her neighbor could do the draining for her. So she hooked up a mechanism that ran from her own roof to the neighbor's roof, then into the neighbor's downspout, and then to the ground, leaving the (paying) neighbor with the full responsibility of doing the draining of two. This wasn't bad (sadomasochistic) enough for her purposes. The system just wasn't working, having been overwhelmed by too much water (e.g., water for two), so as a coup de grâce built out of aggressively over having been rejected, she reported the neighbor to the town's authorities, complaining that her neighbor had an inadequate draining system (i.e., complaining that she didn't have a mechanism with the full capacity for doing the job she was supposed to do, the job for two). Of course, all that was required was two separate drainage systems. The patient denied she was overwhelming the entire system, part of the sadomasochistic denial mechanism found in some borderlines, where the motivation is somewhat paranoid in the sense of blaming and beating up on the second person (the projective "not me" object) for what was the problem of the first person. And she, being herself a lawyer, was able to have her innocent neighbor seriously fined for not providing adequate drainage for her, her neighbor's, own home/roof. Finally, her lawsuit protesting the poor drainage almost wound up with a jail sentence for the innocent neighbor who was distinctly the victim in this case and was rightly refusing to comply on principle and due to the expense.

In any of their calculations, high-level borderlines as a group sadomasochistically ignore or profit by the costs to others and to society of their harshness. Altruism and empathy absent, they expect others to simply absorb the loss and sometimes even take the fall for them without necessarily trying to do better the next time.

Their identity consists of an as-if approach whereby they can easily blend to become someone else not having to maintain their own responsibilities/boundaries. Emotional swings behind attitudinally driven behaviors are also manifestations characteristic of high-level borderlines, leading to a picture of lability and affective unpredictability generally hurtful to others in these individuals' orbit. They can be very nasty so that if you try to give them some advice, they complain "stop trying to run me around and tell me how to live."

Some of them have mood swings, some of which are exogenous; that is, these individuals often get depressed because they feel that they are now getting their comeuppances for the way they have treated other people as the years have gone by. And in some such cases they are right about that. I still feel bad that the suicidal patient referred to throughout didn't accept help; I tried to talk her out of killing herself, but as is characteristic of too many borderlines, she had no intention whatsoever of listening to me, just another person who was eager to run her life for her.

High-level borderlines can be violent too. Certainly the violence part is sadomasochistic in essence because of its relationship between the intense buildup of anger characteristic of these patients and in part because of the disorganization due to the presence of a weak superego that is a characteristic affliction of borderlines on all levels and even of high-level borderlines whose conscience doesn't move in to stop hostile and possibly dangerous behavior toward helpless others.

Chaotic polymorphous perverse infantile sexual and nonsexual disorganization is characteristic only to the extent that it represents a higher level of development and a better prognosis for treatment than for those in which overwhelming primitive aggression has eliminated most possibilities for close meaningful sensual/erotic experience as well as determining the most primitive self-destructive characterological features we expect to be forthcoming from them.

Though there are no good tests for violence and no real way of predicting the possibility of violence to self and/or others, the fortunate thing is that very few of these individuals can be an actual danger to others. Mostly they have spent their strength in ongoing emotional turmoil and now have nothing left to shoot or fire back with, but they can still be potentially "good candidates," should things turn just a little, to shoot up the place, either literally or figuratively, so that those close to them still have to be alert to the possibility that they are getting worse, actually decompensating, and even possibly getting ready to do harm.

Some pathological features of their relationships may be if not qualitatively, then at least quantitatively, different from primitive sadomasochistic interactions in terms of intensity and hence degree of danger prevailing. But too often one end point is the same for all borderlines: loneliness and loss that could have been prevented erodes their lives throughout, leading to isolation that otherwise would not have been necessary, marking the last years of their lives as sad whereby all they can hope for is to enrich their isolation with the maximum of friends and family they can still attract into their low orbit.

Patients with high-level borderline personality organization do not necessarily manifest the chaotic polymorphous perverse infantile sexual and nonsexual behavior that represents a lower level of development and suggests a worse prognosis for treatment. These individuals are often successful personally and occupationally. If politicians, they can still serve their country well; perhaps this is not in spite of but rather because of their borderline condition and with it the insensitivity that keeps them internally goal-directed, focused to the point that they don't really see themselves as the troublemakers that other people think of them as potentially being and as others expect them to actually be and find them.

Psychodynamically, all aspects of borderline issues relate to a more general one: the overall degree to which aggressive realms of early experience (hate) perpetually predominate over early libidinal ones (love) that when combined with a child's possibly innate negative temperament can lead to severe imbalance between oral dependency (masochism) over oral sadism, showing up in a child's prevailing motivation to be a grownup who can successfully devour, control, and strike down others competitively.

In the highest-level borderlines, assertion takes the place of aggression as a consequence of fearfulness. Combining loving and sensual erotic experience with aggression reduces attacks of rage over little to nothing. They also apologize for slippages, helping retain a relationship that they want or need to continue.

To be considered is concern for the patient that involves worry about to what extent his or her function is impaired according to the severity of the manifest psychopathology, which in turn may mainly cause problems with the patient's individual lifestyle and/or those others with whom he or she comes into contact. So, an angry mother might, if herself orally fixated, quash all her daughter's independence over fears of losing her to a husband

and marriage, whereupon the daughter in a rage about being controlled starts cutting herself to mutilate the beauty the mother wants her to not show lest she meet Mr. Right. Most of what we see in the very highest level of borderlines is a retained capacity for sexual enjoyment and minor self-cutting that does not go beyond symbolic self-mutilation (such as lip biting to bleeding, cuticle picking to scarring), both meant to reduce intensity of affect and relieve chronic tension. We might see at most a pathological grandiose self as part of a narcissistic personality organization where the emphasis is on an unconscious triumph over those who try to help and a refusal to willingly submit because of what they see and interpret as being humiliating control ("stop telling me what to do"). An example is the patient who continues to decorate the shared hall of his apartment complex, though this is not the way the tenants are supposed to do things: all have to vote on any changes. This patient showed normal identity formation and the related capacity for object relationships in depth while at the same time avoiding expressing unconscious (hidden) sadism in his criticism of others who did something, even a minor something, that he saw as offending him because it wasn't what he wanted. As Markman says, the gang of different causalities "derives from different sources: as a primitive superego, as an intrusive object related to traumatic experience, as a merger with a powerful persecutory parental figure (or couple) or as a manic part of the self."[4]

9

Classification According to the Level of Psychiatric Illness

The Neurotic and Personality Disorder Spectrum

DEPRESSION

There are sad depressed men and women who make sure they don't have too much fun in their lives. The neurotic level of developmental fixation consists of symptoms that are a compromise formation, the classic product of the typical Freudian tripartite psychic structure of symptom formation. Their angry conflicts around dependency, control, and combat indicate that they are retaining a high level of functioning, with their struggling ultimately being part of normal identity formation as they maintain their display of the related capacity for maintaining good object relationships, those in depth. But unconsciously they struggle to control themselves against the happiness they superficially display, and it is this that soon becomes the dominant core of their characterological features.

On this level sadomasochistic sexual perversions (e.g., cunilinctus or analinctus) and pathological characterological behaviors such as hurtfulness to others, no matter how absent the provocation or what the provocation is, often occur, stand out, and are likely to be the expression of profound unconscious guilt over incestuous and parricidal wishes, with the symptom as such representing a compromise formation simultaneously expressing instinct (anger), guilt (regret), and organizing ego (compromise) such as handcuffing to the bedpost (id) and whipping one's mate (superego) to inflict both pain and pleasure at one and the same time (the compromise formation), then saying "sorry" afterward and trying to make up. In the (psychoanalytic) view, the passivity of masochism itself represents a protection from the dangers of castration ("if I don't assert myself I won't be castrated"). And an unconscious denial of the dangers presented by oedipal rivalry is achieved by the unconscious elimination of all pleasurable sexuality.

At this level of neurotic personality organization, masochistic tendencies tend to be expressed preferentially through self and other-defeating characterological patterns, specifically those that might be collected under the heading of a new clinical entity of "narcissistic (depressive) masochistic personality disorder" as set forth by Cooper.[1] When these individuals are depressed, we see a rise in unconscious superego pressures based especially on excessive restrictions of joy, with self-bashing if one does not live up to one's high moral standards and ethical demands for loving and work, along with expectations that others will do the same. In general, joy vanishes as these patients show excessive superego prohibitions against pleasure, additionally allowing divisive anger at oneself to prevail. As well, they seem to be against the self-gratification characteristic of what most narcissistic-masochistic individuals would be seeking if they allowed themselves to even begin to approach the longing for nirvana that continues to exist somewhere in their unconscious.

When in the manic phase of a bipolar disorder (e.g., as narcissistic neurotic bipolars), these sadomasochists even feel comfortable and fail to complain under conditions when it would be reasonable for them to do so.

Guilt is a significant creative element in masochistic depressive personality disorder, as guilt becomes a major feature in both this personality disorder and in the sadomasochism almost always tied to it. In other words, the relationship between sadomasochism, depression, and guilt is inconvertible and very painful for all concerned.

Not only are the clinical manifestations of depression and sadomasochism overtly similar, but virtually the same unconscious dynamics are also behind each of the behaviors. As a result, a common expression of masochism is depression and a common manifestation of depression is masochism, so that all depression is masochistic and all masochism depressive. When it comes to self-defeat and active hurting of the self, this in part is because unconscious superego pressures leading to excessive self-abusive behaviors such as a high level of worrisomeness and seriousness are characteristic of both disorders. It is hard to distinguish a patient whose life revolves around continually making certain that he or she doesn't do his or her best and another patient who is continually making certain that he or she doesn't deserve to achieve much in life because he or she is unworthy of God's gifts.

The relationship between depression and masochism as put forth by Cooper[2] makes me think of the psychiatrist who was renting me space in his overly large office. While I was on vacation he didn't renew his over-lease on the place and didn't bother to tell me about it, leaving me and my practice nowhere to go when I got back from being away for a month to discover that I no longer had a place to see patients. No amount of his mea culpas seemed sufficient to wash clean the hand that did that dirty deed.

The following are some of the most important points about the relationship between guilt, masochism, and depression:

- Sadism turned toward the self due to guilt becomes masochism. Now the superego, the representation of the frustrating person and of the unacceptable demands of society on the ego, becomes the punishing agency (conscience). The guilt feeling corresponds to the destructive impulse, which comes into conflict with love.
- Guilt is also often related to allowing others to be in control instead of stopping them, which is what one should have done.
- Repressed feelings of guilt lead to a need for suffering.
- Guilt is therapeutic as self-punishment for having behaved in an irrational manner.
- Guilt may involve moral masochism and be a product of negative self-evaluation and the punitive evaluation of others.
- Repressed feelings of guilt leading to a need for suffering make guilt welcome because it is felt to be deserved retribution.
- Guilt is a moral stance involving the feeling that violations must be balanced by retribution and that transgressions must be balanced by pain.
- Developmentally, guilt starts with real (unavoidable) transgressions by the child against the parents; these transgressions are unavoidable given the nature of events related to growing up. Therefore, appropriate as well as inappropriate guilt predictably develops and is carried along into adulthood directed toward old and new (parental) transference figures. Guilt in this way grows developmentally (e.g., guilt may come from one's evolving relationship with one's parents). Can the child ever avoid doing things that inevitably elicit guilt on his or her part because of the innately very childish nature of childish acts?
- Guilt involves self-recriminations for prior sins; in the form of self-recrimination it can take numerous interchangeable forms (e.g.,

a paranoid vendetta against all concerned versus hysterical temper tantrums such as throwing all of one's finest possessions out of the house and onto the lawn).

- Guilt sometimes but not always arises predominately from within implicitly. But a range of real-life guilt-inducing events can give rise to guilt (e.g., the guilt associated with moral masochism can arise out of being preached to, resulting in a reactive, not an endogenous, depression). Rejection by others becomes a source of guilt if the individual thinks "what did I do to deserve this?" Treatment implications are obvious.
- Also eliciting guilt is oneself not being nice to others due to resentment manifest as rejecting others. This of course adds to one's own rage over having been thwarted by others when one is trying to unselfishly pursue a meaningful relationship with them.
- Severity of the guilt is one factor leading to choosing real as distinguished from merely emotional punishments; additionally, comorbidity determines the style of guilty retaliatory behaviors (e.g., *paranoid* vendettas vs. *hysterical* temper tantrums). These self-recriminations can substitute one for the other. What is not entirely known is why cutting oneself might be specifically chosen over other methods of atonement. For example, comorbidity determines the specific style of guilty sadomasochistic behavior indulged in.
- How the parents respond to a child's behavior counts too. For example, ostracizing children via passivity toward their plights, making insufficient effort to care when a child is suffering, and failing to offer reassurance that what you, my child, did wasn't so bad after all (so don't feel so bad about it) are specific guilt-inducing behaviors/cognitions vis-à-vis the very young and even the somewhat older child. Calling upon the superego to step in can ultimately be a good thing.
- Unresolved conflicts over the experience and expression of specific emotional needs (e.g., one's anger toward one's parents) have lasting effects, and guilt pertains whether or not the anger toward oneself/others is justified. Putting one's parents in a nursing home for one's convenience, in effect abandoning them there, is a powerful guilt inducer.
- Many different actions are aimed at achieving relief from self-recrimination. Clearly sadomasochism isn't the only manifestation of/way to deal with guilt. One can absent oneself from one's victims in the realization that if the victim is present, the guilt is intensified. Other substitute ways, mostly symbolic, for guilty behavior are available to sadomasochists. In turn, guilt may not lead to (i.e., is not always handled by) sadomasochistic reparative techniques.

- Not being helpful enhances guilt. An example: an individual is being beaten up and robbed at an ATM machine; strangers pass by without seeming to notice it. A recent story of the cop who was being attacked by others trying to get his gun and no passers-by did anything but take his picture is another example. In sum, guilt may not lead to (i.e., is not always handled by) sadomasochism. People often deal with their guilt about having been bad not masochistically but instead by being extra good (e.g., doing a good deed). This is the dynamic of some altruists. For these individuals, helping victims of others' misdeeds might be the best possible way to make amends without increasing one's own guilty thoughts and hence enhancing one's guilty behavior.
- A principle hypothesis of the role that depression plays in masochism is the depressive oedipal belief that in no way do I compare to my father, occurring in the context of a generally high level of functioning, an identity formation that is intact (one knows for certain who one is), and a retention of the capacity for solid object relationships at least in some settings (and therefore no relief in these abandonments).
- In both depression and masochism, guilt is expressed in the excessive criticism of and efforts to control oneself and others. Here deliberate efforts to be nice to other people if misapplied excessively paradoxically makes others feel guilty, and this boomerangs.
- Unconscious (sadistic) efforts to control others are in actuality expressed through the induction of feelings of guilt in others, one of the sadomasochist's most striking/dominant characterological features (talents).
- Prominent also is an excessive fear of being criticized for self-affirmative behavior ("Boy, who do you think you are?") especially when combined with a harsh, critical tendency toward others due to unconscious identification with one's own superego attitudes toward/demands of others.
- These latter themes mostly occur in the context of a generally high level of functioning, normal identity formation, and retention of the related capacity for object relationships in depth.
- Well-defined conflicts may be absent in psychotic or borderline sadomasochists whose structure is less imposing than otherwise because their superego doesn't rule, for those with psychotic tendencies are mainly disorganized due to the harsh weight of disparate forces all demanding discharge at once.
- Guilt is often related to allowing others to have their way instead of setting limits on them when that's what one should have done and feel regretful about not having done.

- Guilt is therapeutic self-punishment that provides closure to one's self-evaluation as to how one has previously behaved, perhaps especially relative to one's sexuality. Of course, a price must then be paid for feeling guilty, and there is guilt over not being able to stop feeling guilty.

CYCLOTHYMIA PERSONALITY DISORDER ORGANIZATION

In cyclothymia, the general chaos of interpersonal relationships, the combination of clinging dependency and aggressive reactions in the context of presumed or actual rejection, creates chaotic love relations also characteristic of (higher-level) borderline patients. In these milder (relational?) sadomasochistic primitive narcissistic patients there is a display of an incapacity to fall very deeply in love, with the presence of transitory infatuations repeatedly followed by devaluation of the love object. One forms many in-groups that, however, shift frequently in their constitution due to inherent interpersonal conflicts arising within the group. Narcissistic forms of sexual promiscuity may coexist (e.g., notching one's gun to feel good about oneself and displaying oneself sexually to others in orgy rooms), and pride about one's accomplishments replaces love for one's objects. This process can be hardly distinguishable from sadomasochistic sexual promiscuity in which potentially gratifying love relationships are undermined and destroyed for a momentary sexual thrill often involving some forms of paraphilia. Sometimes the patient settles into a forever stable but clearly sadomasochistic relationship, often with another narcissistic or sadomasochistic love object.

However enmeshed they are in the midst of such chaos, cyclothymic sadomasochistic patients may still have the capacity to fall in some form of love, establish deep and dependent even if clinging relationships, and evince a greater potential for stability of love relations than chaotic borderlines and primitive narcissistic patients, whose manifest capabilities frequently are or at least seem to be (but are fundamentally not necessarily) much better than that of the cyclothymic individual. In ongoing so-called committed relationships sexual cheating is common, and in those with a great deal of disposable cash, payments for silence so as not to wreck one's marriage are not unheard of.

HISTRIONIC PERSONALITY DISORDER ORGANIZATION

In their nature there is envy of others that leads to criticizing them in order to devalue them and make them seem less of a threat. There is also a success phobia that leads to a failure to make the best use of important opportunities for success and happiness in their own lives. Deserving but fearing success, they challenge themselves only to fail most or all challenges. Failure leads to self-pity as they convince others such as their therapists of the hopelessness of their situation (with self-pity dynamically speaking equal to a sense of submission to their own superego ideal). There is a compensatory tendency to deny one's own failures by beating up on others, deflating them comparatively in order to rescue at least some sense of success of their own to counter their generalized sense of self-disapproval. Defensive histrionic tirades are common in politics and should be read as "you, my competition, is the defective one." In fact, the entire country sometimes seems run by primitive histrionic opposition against leaders who are imperfect but in their own (histrionic) way effective overall.

Guilt is strong and has many sources for these patients, the most common one cited being oedipal guilt consisting of unconscious guilt over oedipal longings, leading to their repression and expression in fantasy only followed by self-punishment as a response to guilt over their dimly recognized incestuous oedipal strivings that keep trying to get through.

They have many somatic symptoms, and these represent physical punishments for repressed oedipal fantasies, the classic example being the paralyzed arm as a self-punishment for sexual desires.

Histrionic sadomasochists display considerable anxiety around both attachment and distancing. Histrionic sadomasochists go through life holding on to the early dualistic view of people as being all bad or all good, without compromise. When their loving feelings emerge, they become anxious about others taking over their lives and hurt the object to disentangle themselves from him or her; when their angry aggressive feelings emerge, they become afraid of closeness and go into their distancing mode catalyzed by sadistic feelings urging them to destroy the objects they feel might be doing them harm (specifically by enveloping them unmercifully). These are mother and father transferences that later are to emerge and persist as transference to almost everybody (e.g., to the therapist as well as to someone they just met over the Internet), revealing a great deal about the histrionic sadomasochistic syndrome itself but too often usually without necessarily advancing the cause of developing and sustaining healthy object relationships or succeeding in treatment, should they go for help.

As a consequence, they display a degree of ambivalence toward their objects consisting of the familiar "go away, come back, I love you" mixed feelings about enmeshment and distancing.

In a masochistic phase, they are reluctant to abandon even especially troublesome objects even though, or just because, it hurts to hold on to people who behave negatively toward them, yet these are the only people they really like and feel comfortable with. As a friend said about a dyadic relationship with someone who has been treating a mutual friend harshly,

"I don't like the way she made your life hell with her unstable moods and her lashing out."

In contrast, in the sadistic phase they are eager to lash out unpredictably, often provoked by some minor issue having to do with a failure they feel they are accused of, a closeness they cannot tolerate, and/or others' controlling ways meant to be helpful but that they feel are excessive or conversely lacking in some respect or (paradoxically) being too intrusive and taking over their lives, as if they are forced to follow them. As a grandiose narcissistic patient said when told to consider paying attention to an attractive man's romantic advances, "Nobody like you tells me what to do."

Anxiety is also found around issues of aggression; these involve anger over deprivation, over having too little, the wrong kind of, or not enough control in specific situations; competitive anger, whereby one loses in situations as two or more people struggle for the same prize-over feeding (preoedipal) issues, toilet training issues (preoedipal), and oedipal issues, all taking center stage as events that remain continuously significant due to having been retained from childhood in somewhat of their original form.

PASSIVE-AGGRESSIVE PERSONALITY DISORDER ORGANIZATION

One of the most sadistic of disorders, in fact one predicated on sadism to others, is passive-aggression. The *trait* of passive-aggression describes a behavior without referencing a full *disorder.* As a trait, passive-aggression is universally accepted as a formulation describing a discrete behavior/behavioral constellation that few if any observers deny exists, admitting that passive-aggressive personality traits are common in the real world, where they are in fact universal, having become manifest as hurtful interpersonal transactions of a given negative specificity consisting of sneaky anger. These interventions disturb the lives of others and occasionally one's own life and not infrequently even end life prematurely. A common example of a sadomasochistic passive-aggressive trait might be hurtful obstructionism via the practice of excessive immobility consisting of a refusal to be rational when one is asked to "move it."

Here too, important dynamic considerations apply in differentiating one trait from another, for obstructionism due to obsessive-compulsive personality disorder vacillation resulting from uncertainty is not the same thing and so doesn't have the same diagnostic implication as obstructionism due to suppressed anger toward others. As is notable, the trait of stubbornness can be put down either to a lack of effort due to laziness or to purposeful resistance.

NARCISSISTIC PERSONALITY DISORDER ORGANIZATION

I use the term "narcissism" to describe the trait of self-indulgence and self-love (e.g., "he is an egoist") and to refer to the dynamics involving a developmental stage predating the stage of mature object love, that is, to the dynamics of the narcissistic trait, and in a diagnostic sense to refer either to a personality disorder in its own right (narcissistic personality disorder) or to an aspect of another disorder such as the narcissism found in schizophrenia, borderline personality disorder, and depression (e.g., the licking of one's wounds found in depressed masochistic individuals who go over and over how hurt they have been and how hurt they feel even now by a world that disdains, ignores, and brutalizes them).

A certain degree of narcissism is normal. It is inherent in self-awareness (thinking a lot about oneself and sometimes mainly or only of oneself) and in the sense of elevated self-worth.

The following will illustrate some specifics as to how the pathological narcissism of sadomasochism can be hurtful to self and others; some clinical characteristic behaviors of both normal and pathological narcissism that end up damning, insulting, or failing to support and otherwise being hurtful to self and/or others are described. A purpose of what follows is to stress the overlap between narcissism/narcissistic personality disorder and sadomasochism/sadomasochistic personality disorder: that is, how both cover similar or the same territory in important aspects and so can be difficult to tell apart.

Almost all observers agree that narcissistic personality traits are part of the matrix of sadomasochism, where they become manifest as interpersonal transactions of a given self-oriented specificity. The narcissistic personality traits central to be used in the service of sadomasochism have in this context a panoply of special meanings mostly implying overconcern for the individual manifesting them. For example, sadomasochistic obstructionism is here a way to convey hostility, a manifestation of the seeking of selfish personal gain (via retention of something valuable to the sadistic individual's needs) and sadomasochistic vacillation (not giving one's all but instead holding back by being unreliable as a way to retain something for oneself in a selfishness without parallel in other neurosis).

Conversely, because of the commonality of narcissistic personality traits, the diagnosis of sadomasochistic personality disorder from one or a few narcissistic personality traits should not be made unless a high concentration of traits exist in any one person and the dynamics associated with these traits are associated in some way with sadomasochistic intent.

Characteristic of narcissistic traits embedded in sadomasochism are the following: inordinate self-pride, overwhelming self-concern, ideas of perfection with a simple reluctance to accept blame or criticism (in some ways itself narcissistically resembling that which arises out of paranoid projection that cleanses the self of any measure of responsibility by blaming others), an absence of altruism so that what appears instead is an empathy deficit (this may be due to projective identification whereby one misinterprets the intentions/needs of others according to what is really an empathy substitute, since an understanding of what others might need is really based on what one needs oneself), and a grandiosity leading to errors of judgment that can look hypomanic, often presenting itself, as does hypomania, as lack of concern for another's feelings and well-being.

A degree of specialness/inordinate self-pride. A simple example is supplied by a man who was inordinately proud of his handmade shoes that were, however, plain to the point of unstylishness. Yet he believed his shoes to be "the finest in New York," them having made him sufficiently distinctive to stand out from the rest. When he was a baby his mother was proud of his little outfits that made him the best-dressed baby on the block, while anyone who disagreed with her and ignored his specialness was roundly savaged for being insufficiently appreciative of how the child, like her and his shoes, stood out from the rest. In a short time, the child came to believe that he too stood out from the crowd, and any opinion to the contrary ran counter to the child's self-view as an object admittedly able to gain attention and kudos from the plebes. In fact, the child himself became quite nasty when others didn't appear to be sufficiently informed about and appreciative of his specialness, with temper tantrums invading relationships if the possibility that this was the perfect child, one any mother would be happy to display to any of the neighbors, was not recognized.

A high level of self-concern. A most obvious quality of the sadomasochistic narcissist is inordinate self-concern, what laymen perceive as simple egocentricity. This quality is manifest in a tendency to exaggerate the importance of one's experiences and feelings and to see events of equal or lesser relevance to others in a highly personal, excessively significant light. The endless baby picture show symbolizes this aspect of narcissism on the part of both the mother and the child, who likely senses that he or she is on display quite beyond where boundaries of propriety ought to come into play, and ultimately the child ought to figuratively stop desperately blowing on his or her nails, wiping them for shine, and polishing them on the fabric of his or her outer garment for luster.

Ideas of absolute perfection. Less obvious than these traits but equally significant is a characteristic reluctance to accept blame or criticism that seems to lurk in all child-to-adult sadomasochistic interactivity and is reminiscent of the extroversion of the bad me that takes place in paranoia. The sadistic "tu quoque" or "you're one too" and "nobody's as perfect as I" infantile argument, starting at remarkably young ages in some cultural groups and extending to bullying of others (often for trends that one doesn't admire in oneself), is characteristic of the more paranoid subcultures we see in today's society, where children are involved as central enough and are believed to be as excessively impressive enough to be impressed by their own self-worth.

A patient wishes to have a big mausoleum when she dies. She says that "I want my dogs put in there with me." I asked a reasonable question: "Does that mean you are going to euthanize your dogs and have them cremated with you?" She bursts into a fury at me: "What kind of dunce do you think I am?" As it turns out, she is referring to urns of ashes from her previous dogs. But how am I to know this unless she tells me? That is why I asked; now, I know something I didn't know before. How is this a bad thing?

Absence of altruism/failure of empathy, however gestures of such may be made for the sake of appearance, as happens with her, is as reflective of what happens in some politically oriented societies representing the narcissist's all too characteristic lack of concern about and focus on others and, in this individual as I knew her, likely reflective of a true deficit of empathy. In the more insightful narcissist, we find either a real-appearing empathy that is, however, compensatory, or real-appearing empathic gestures that in fact consist of projective identification whereby others are congratulated for having qualities that one finds in oneself, and one interprets the needs of others incorrectly strictly according to one's own needs and how well they are identified and satisfied in the persona of others according to one's own views. Thus, one man, aware that his self-preoccupation deprived a woman of love, expected to make it up to her with compensating gifts but failed to do so because via projective identification, he chooses gifts more for himself than for her, and she naturally was aware of it. For example, soon after she discussed her bad feet with him (his father was a podiatrist), for her Xmas gift he gave her a nice and expensive but rather pedestrian pair of cuticle scissors.

Bullying is narcissistic, for it says "you're defective in ways I secretly feel I am defective, and I recognize it all too well and criticize you to punish you for being that way, just to make you more aware of your flaws, the very ones I condemn in myself." (A bully is often a child who, having fully identified with his or her parents, treats other children the way his or her parents treated him and now seeks and often gets an audience for his or her own parental rage.)

Grandiosity. Here egocentricity reaches massive proportions leading to errors of judgment of a hypomanic sort, as when a mother enters a toddler in a beauty pageant for which the child is hardly qualified, causing the child serious self-questioning because he or she has been put into a situation that is so foreign to the child's nature that no good can possibly come of it. Such children have been known to become seriously depressed and eat themselves up alive over their supposed incompetence, which is, however, not incompetency, not their fault, and not due to something they lack but instead is due to an incontrovertible absence of readiness for a certain role they are being asked to play but are not yet ready for biologically, physically, or emotionally. Their sadomasochism in return is a rebellion to show their displeasure by treating themselves as defective and letting their parents know that they are being made to feel that way through parental lack of considerateness and/or neglect.

Motivations/objectives that are self-oriented in the extreme are common and often lead to outlandish behaviors. Grace DeBell, a psychoanalyst in the 1960s, would give as her favorite example of such behavior the woman who pulled up for her first and only analytic appointment scantily dressed, hair dyed blond, in a very expensive, showy convertible, only to be announcing her arrival 15 minutes early by blasting her "see me now I'm here" horn and, because her session was delayed, indulged in annoying attention-seeking behaviors by loudly revving up the car as if to say "What are you waiting for? I'm ready."[3]

In *oral* narcissism the objective is demanded nourishment both figuratively and literally, in *anal* narcissism the objective is assuming power (for me and rarely/ever for you), and in *phallic* narcissism the objective is sexual conquest (notching one's guns to indicate how many rare specimens one has brought down from the earth and skies, with an element of the conquest annoying when forced upon others involuntarily, because these others may not care for a person who brags that he or she collects the skins of wild animals).

One characteristic of such individuals is that they don't have that much interest in what you have to say about yourself. In fact, not even waiting for you to finish saying it, they hurtfully overwhelmingly talk over your productions as if you count for little, sadistically making others in the room feel bad as if, compared to me, they have little or nothing to contribute to the discussion. Here too as in sadomasochistic borderlines, we see the relative incapacity to fall in love due to much of the love by now already spoken for, its having already been plastered on the self. Paradoxically, we sometimes see excessively intense falling in love, the opposite of distancing, characterized as "I am already falling in love; now all I need is the person to express my feelings about." Associated is the belief that "I am so great that nobody would not want me." This can lead the sadist to force his or her intentions on the masochist.

As with borderlines, with whom narcissists often overlap, we see the presence of transitory infatuations alternating with repeated expected devaluation of the love object due to a "gimme more" mentality that especially blossoms when an object doesn't perform cooperatively as expected. This is often marked by off-putting narcissistic forms of interpersonal selfishness whereby the sadism is prominent over the masochism, and in fact the masochism fades into the background except as a reaction to the loss, one to be inevitably expressed in the form of victim retaliation.

We often find that kind of sexual promiscuity where little thought is given to what attracts you to me in favor of only considering what I find attractive about you, so that even an unpleasant sexually harassing man is able to convince himself that though women complain, they really like to be groped no matter how much they protest. This is hardly distinguishable from masochistic sexual promiscuity in which potentially gratifying love relationships are inevitably undermined and destroyed because objects have been initially selected one after the other without any regard for the needs and desires of the object and the desirability of the person sadomasochistically forcing himself on the other person in the dyad. Truly unappealing personages feel that they make suitable love objects even for the most desirable of other people, who supposedly don't know what they are missing. Often stalking is the result.

Often the sadist settles into a stable but clearly self-serving destructive sadomasochistic relationship with another who is him or herself a narcissistic individual chosen to be the other object in a dyad. Hurtfulness emerges to others from one's own desires being so all-encompassing and excessive that the victim feels consumed and reacts in a way that disappointment in the party of the first part is inevitable. The other person is seen as being desperate for love and unwilling to give up the few crumbs of a relationship that rarely come his or her way: the object should feel lucky enough to have been selected for any form of attention. One-way dimensionality due to the first person's selfishness/self-concern and lack of real feeling for the object prevails.

The negative responses on the part of others are integrated not by an appeal to the need for sacrifice of the one who is the victim in the case but instead by intimidation and manipulation to gain the sadist's ends, with devaluation of others coming naturally out of overvaluing the ability of the self to gain his or her ends no matter how much at the expense of the other person in the affair. The guiding light illuminates the slogan "Who cares about you?"

Narcissistic masochists in forming these often one-way relationships with another, the designated patsy, often select initially unavailable or potentially frustrating objects, which means that there is a typical longing on their part for partners who are desperate. The lip service involves mutuality, but the reality here is that there is one-way intimidation, so that for a relationship to work one member at least has to accept the relationship as it is and tolerate the destructive features in the relationship that forms, accepting the fact that there is a price to pay for the survival of the relationship on the whole. That is, one of the two people in a dyad has to be willing to forgo some gratification and accept some deprivation just to form the relationship and keep things going. What is frequent is the breakdown of relationships when both of the members of the dyad are severely narcissistic. Now the relationship becomes a struggle between equals, and the usual struggle is over who deserves and gets the most out of this.

Of course, when self-sacrifice in the service of perpetuating a less than ideal relationship along the lines of "any relationship is better than none" and "this one isn't perfect but it's not so bad after all" occurs, it may reflect a mature emotional disposition that implies a creative/altruistic adaptation/contribution on the part of one or both members of the dyad. Suffering in the service of some legitimate (ego-syntonic bilateral) goal is, while uncommon, not unhealthy unless it comes down to the tyrannical suppression of the other in the service of achieving one's own goals—advanced regardless of what others want and think solely to fulfill personal needs. It is unfortunate if it comes down to the sadistic narcissist grasping an advantage to oneself at the expense of another.

Most times narcissistic superego pressures are unconscious and need to be freed from repression so that all concerned can see what is happening. Psychopathic sadomasochism where one member of a dyad deliberately goes after what one wants even though it is at the expense of another has no place in long-term relationships, where one party is constantly forced to face the ongoing fear of being misused/abandoned.

Sadomasochism embedded in a narcissistic personality organization displays patterns where overt functioning frequently seems to be much better (e.g., admirable than it should at least theoretically seem to be). This is partly because our society condones a lot of both sadomasochism and narcissism, and therefore the combination calls little attention to itself even for those looking for pathological behavior, or the behavior actually elicits a prideful social response (in some societies). This said, narcissistic sadomasochism is still me-focused due to interest for the self, subsumed under concern for the other. Some people stay together the more properly to get close enough to really hate each other.

10

Classification According to the Level of Psychiatric Illness

Post-Traumatic Stress Disorder

An ongoing question is this: Is the unrelenting pursuit of misery the product of developmental trauma, for example, the result of the behavior of punitive or neglectful, subjugating or humiliating, caregivers? Or does it reflect a particular temperamental vulnerability or failure of resilience of ego structures and self-organization? (According to Ferenczi, "masochism . . . is pleasurably obeying, and this one learns in childhood from one's parents.")[1]

Sadomasochism is in part the product of phase-specific psychological developmental problems, many of which are related to early traumatic experiences. Thus, the neglected very young child might already feel traumatized by being ignored and develop a marasmic depression (one characterized by severe withdrawal and abject sadness) associated with abandonment fears, leading the child to give up on relationships, retreat into him or herself, and become lonely and isolated as self-punishment.

One way to organize our thinking about childhood traumas and our thinking about their effects in adult life is according to the traumas being ones of omission or commission. The mother or father either doesn't respond by joining in the applause for the child's latest musical adventure. Or the mother or father predictably become abusive to the child, say, by spanking him or her for behavioral deviations that count for little or nothing, doing so just on a principle of some unjust philosophical nature.

Classification is thus according to where the child is developmentally when significant trauma occurs. Furthermore, developmental phases interact with characteristic traumas associated with each developmental phase (e.g., excessive control marring healthy anality involving issues of traumatic potty training).

Mostly childhood psychic development can be divided into three phases, with characteristic traumas associated with each one of these phases leading to specific pathognomonic sadomasochistic behavioral patterns later in life.

Oral-level abusive traumatization. This occurs in the realm of inadequate caretaking. This actually fosters dependency by depriving the child of that which he or she needs as a toddler; the child never gets enough care and so goes through life always wanting more, making the child into a needy adult always looking for someone to be dependent on. In this realm of oral level traumatization/abuse, self-induced deprivation later becomes a masochistic lifestyle so that children criticized and punished for being excessively demanding when they express any needs of their own, however legitimate, for love and attention come to misinterpret their normal needs as excessive neediness. Such boys and girls forevermore hide in the shadows of deliberately induced painful active personal deprivation to avoid feeling the worse pain of overwhelming unpredictable rejection/loss at the hands of others. They become overly passive, accepting, and self-denying adults out of a fear that complaining and standing up for themselves will be counterproductive, since they come to believe that this will certainly lead to the rupture of even tentative relationships, ones they hold on to for dear life, and so need and want more of than anything else. All concerned become hypersensitive to being chastised. Such children deprive themselves of close committed relationships to avoid being blamed and punished for a relationship ending should it not work out.

Anal-level abuse traumatization. This often takes the form of excessively rigid controlling regimentation along the lines of "this and only this is the right way to do things." This creates an ongoing submissive child whose masochism reflects the constant cry not of "I need more love" but rather "I need cooperation, understanding, and advice," not of "I need adequate attention along the lines of 'care for me, please, you see how deprived I feel and am,'" but rather along opposite lines, whereby "I need to be left alone"—in the latter case the original traumatic abuse having taken the form either of excessive supervision (or possibly a paradoxical absence of appropriate active organizing feedback by parents who let the child run too wild for the good of all concerned). The result: the parents have created a masochistic child who feels invisible and so wouldn't think twice about running away from home, or its equivalent, even without the slightest provocation.

Also in the realm of anal-level traumas, parents criticize a child's normal rebelliousness, leaving the child being excessively passive as the only alternative to being healthfully assertive, always disavowing aspirations by self-abnegating. These children become masochistic because they equate growing up freely with being put down/imprisoned. They become masochistic to avoid standing up to the people who try to regiment them and instead yield to people who act like their bosses when they are in fact equals or even underlings, the child acting passive out of a fear, reasonable or not, of saying something that will be antagonistic to someone. Masochism is here protective by helping suppress dangerous antagonistic sadistic wishes.

Excessive or inadequate *phallic-level* abuse doesn't take the form of lack of support/lack of input of love or of specific excessive abuse/inadequate control around such issues as cleanliness and orderliness but instead involves being put down for assertion, attempted serious competition, budding masculine sexuality in boys, or in women for wanting equality (e.g., to be less passive and more active, not just there as part of the scenery). The culture tells women to be inactive; they can now only protest via the forms of sadomasochistic equivalents available to them, especially that of a passive-aggressive nature.

Also in the realm of phallic-level traumas, emerging sexuality is chastised, particularly when oedipal trends are prominent, leaving masochism as a way to avoid dangerous sexual competitiveness with parental figures. Punitive castration anxiety is dealt with by preventive anticipatory (masochistic) self-castration (ultimately creating a disorder with features of avoidant personality disorder).

Traumatic sibling rivalry, often left out of the picture of traumatic developmental insults as presented, leads to feelings of being too successfully competitive lest one get ganged up on by favored brothers and sisters. It almost always involves the boy's sensitivity to being emasculated by the other boys and girls in the family. Indeed, a boy's sexuality is often more overt and so more available to be overtly criticized than a girl's, leaving boys more open to criticism and hence castration anxiety/symbolic castration.

It would appear that more boys become masochistically defensive throughout their lives than do girls; that is, boys become more self-apologetic for their native physicality than do girls, leaving them, as they see it, more vulnerable, having to find ways to better handle displays of shame and guilt that envelop their sexuality. Thus, in one scheme in matters phallic, masochism is a defense, and sadism is a breakthrough to get past the defense ("I'll show you. You can't treat me this way.").

Thus, for both boys and men and for girls and women adult sexuality, which ought to consist of both healthy conflict-free phallic and genital components, is connected to ideas of punishment for being defective, often due to having become excessive.

When it comes to sexuality, a connection between the physical (what is right to do) and the moral (what is right to think) makes both of these dangerous, surrounded by forbidden aspects. All that is left is a failure to thrive and prosper in terms of morality and physical sexuality, leaving sadomasochistic object choices as one of the only possible outcomes for satisfying exchanges/discharge. Shame becomes the handmaiden of sexuality and is often a guiding component of the few actual thoughts and behaviors that occur (manage to get through) in the sexual sadomasochist, to the point that even mentioning scientific details about sexuality got one of my medical books banned from one website. Beating oneself or another (for the same behavior that one desires or acts on) is then a way to handle the secret shame over being beaten for taking pleasure in the warmth and love of another's body. A boy who shows his sister his vows that he will never do anything like that again can go on to become an adult who has only secret affairs or, what too often naturally follows, rarely seeks sex at all, and when he does have sexual contact he is not satisfied and is barely able to enjoy it. Or, as with many patients with post-traumatic stress disorder, he or she repeats unsatisfactory activity as part of a repetition compulsion to make things come out satisfactorily once and for all or to be sure that they don't come out wrong all over again. Too, such children when punished for something (almost anything) else in actuality really feel punished for their sexuality, leading to what is essentially the same outcome: the linkage between sexuality on all levels and being punished for any and all wishes that can be (mis)interpreted as sexual.

Sadomasochism is then both a way to avoid and a way to express one's assertiveness and sexuality. And certain aspects of sadistic sexuality, particularly rape and forceful paraphilias, remain the only way that individuals, overpowering another for pleasure, can themselves ever enjoy sexual pleasure without an aspect of guilt associated with what should be normal God-given behavior. Some individuals conclude that sex is only for procreation (and sometimes not even that) and otherwise should be held in abeyance lest one become a "sinner man."

To conclude, clearly sadomasochism is often connected with sexual behavior as much as with aggressive behavior. Too, in the public eye, anything but missionary-position sexuality is sadomasochistic, and the two, aggressiveness and sexuality, become intimately intertwined. As a result, too many men and women tend to develop psychoneuroses with prevailingly post-traumatic sadomasochistic features, among which are depression, obsessive-compulsive personality disorder, narcissism, and histrionic personality disorder, four of the numerous emotional disorders most intimately connected with post-traumatic sadomasochism due to the prominence of early psychological/traumatic developmental problems, with the post-traumatic features associated with dependency, control, and assertion.

Some sexual sadists can become violent to others, while other (many) moral and sexual masochists relinquish pleasure entirely rather than express any of their needs and can only enjoy themselves in private, having activating uncorporeal fantasies. They punish themselves and make sure certain others will also punish them for being too demanding, competitive, or overly preoccupied with being morally activated and physically active. They often repeat the scenario of early traumatic abuse with a series of adult substitutive abusers and additionally become enmeshed pathologically with abusive people and maintain these enmeshments even at great cost and self-sacrifice. They seek out and tolerate those who abuse them in an attempt to master their early traumatic experiences through repetition; maybe this time things will come out right, the futile hope that this time things will turn out better because this abuser will be different from the rest, and he or she will come around and treat them more kindly (i.e., less sadomasochistically). These attempts to seek a reversal of post-traumatic fortune exist mainly or only in situations where a changeover is quite unlikely to occur, simply because the individuals involved seek it from the very people who are most like their early abusers, and therefore attempts to continue relationally with them, being predictably failures, only prolong and fixate the inner sense of badness and hopelessness.

AGGRESSION

All of these phases—oral sadistic, anal sadistic, and phallic sadistic—are in turn associated with their particular brand of aggression. The introduction of aggression into the developmental pattern of all these phases highlights the relationships between early developmental events and the onset and nature of sadomasochism involving the child feeling aggressive for

- having been ignored and not cared for;
- wanting to rebel against the absence of supervision for those who feel they are being insufficiently managed and lack longed-for reasonable regimentation; they feel they are floundering because nobody wants to guide them (which to them means that nobody is out there listening to them; and
- feelings of frustrated self-expression and power seeking.

Fixation and regression become significant, with stress at one phase often creating regression to an earlier phase, one where the child felt safer and has already accomplished a degree of mastery.

As a result, many men and women tend to develop ordinary psychoneuroses with prevailingly post-traumatic and sadomasochistic features. Pounding hysterical headaches are by some seen as combined sexual and aggressive discharge and punishment alike for sexual enjoyment as well as constituting symptoms that often seem to be more complaints directed at others ("You give me a headache") than pure manifestations of personal suffering.

Some traumatized sadists can become violent, but most do not. Instead, they punish themselves and make certain others will also punish them, but they at most become annoying.

In conclusion, developmental phases—oral, anal, and phallic—are therefore associated with their particular brand of aggression. The introduction of aggression into the developmental pattern of all these phases highlights the relationships between early developmental events and the onset of sadomasochism, which is basically a disorder involving problems with the metabolism of aggression fused with issues of a moral and sexual nature further enhanced by issues related to problems with object relationships.

11

Various Motivations for Being a Sadomasochist

In this chapter I discuss what is motivating these individuals to act as they do toward other people along the lines of what he must have been thinking just now to behave that way and what she is trying to say to me that I do or don't necessarily want to hear.

The literature emphasizes that the main psychological function of masochism is that it is a way of avoiding uncontrollable suffering by willingly undertaking other milder, more controllable suffering.

But not all sadomasochistic behaviors are reducible to their elemental parts (e.g., that which motivates them). Some, like cutting oneself, appear to be more in the nature of primary drives that are in the present state of our knowledge irreducible into their component parts. Only some behaviors can, like other neurotic behaviors, be profitably understood from the point of view of the Freudian tripartite formation of symptoms.

AS AN AVOIDANCE OF SHAME

Some try to hide how sadomasochistic they are. For them, self-abuse and being abusive to others is not something to be proud of. They care if they look good in public; otherwise, they will or won't go outside (e.g., on some days they can be seen wearing certain articles of clothing that are not in style, though on others they are the epitome of stylishness, trying to impress others with how chic they are and how much better they are than you).

In particular, because masochism = secret shame, issues of basic trust often come up and are put to the test: for example, will you keep my destructive behavior secret from others who don't need to know what I am like or up to, or will you rat on me about some very private matter that I confided to you? The question becomes, can I trust you to not go too far in telling others about what I really want, who I really am, and prove to me that you will not betray and humiliate me by giving away my secret fantasies? There is an exchange involved: if you keep my behavior secret from others who don't need to know, I will never rat on some of the things you don't want to be known about you.

TO LET OTHERS KNOW EXACTLY HOW YOU FEEL AS A SADOMASOCHIST (MASOCHISM AS A SOURCE OF PROSELYTIZING)

Some sadomasochists deal with their secret shame by denying who they really are. They are ashamed about being the way they are, and instead of explaining what they do and why they do it, they keep their thoughts to themselves to hide their real identity. Others don't mind showing and telling what they stand for and how proud they are of what they do, so they give themselves a vote of confidence and act accordingly. Two ideas in particular seem to mystify most people looking in on sadomasochists: all human life is built on striving to decrease suffering and pain, yet sadomasochists do just the reverse; and it is women who constitute the majority of the human race and are the most masochistic, which means that fundamentally many more women than men are out to seek pain and suffering. Both ideas frequently meet with skepticism and often with overt opposition.

Some sadomasochists wish to involve other (not necessarily sadistic and masochistic) individuals in their lives to the max; in such cases it almost appears as if they are advocating sadomasochism. Activist groups are particularly adept at this and proud of the results, if any. Almost no one advocates obsessive-compulsive disorder, but the opposite is the case with sadomasochism, which seeks to enroll other advocates along the same lines.

We can learn a lot that is useful about how sadomasochists operate if we just listen to sadomasochistic men and women speak without interrupting their tales of woe and anger. Hopefully, the reason they think and act the way they do is to look ahead to other solutions potentially available to them and others like them. But most look back to old problems as they focus on what they could have done that they didn't do: resentments about how others caused them to make mistakes and could-a's and should-a's about roads not taken, relieving pent-up interpersonal tensions of yesterday with old often hapless victims of today and even advising us as to how to live our own lives along the routes they have chosen for themselves that may not work for either them or us.

Proselytizing has a narcissistic function for some, closely related to know-it-all omnipotence. Sadomasochists tend to be too forceful about how and why others should live like them. They are effectively acting out aggressive fantasies of complete domination of self and others, often refusing to give up until others follow their leads, sometimes desolately.

Many masochistic and sadistic individuals wish to involve other (sadistic and masochistic) individuals in their lives on a day-to-day basis. Hoping to do so effectively, they spread the various words in circulation about the value of sadomasochism and how they are actually proud of being advocates of pain for themselves and others. Example are the principle that the lower they go the lower we go and the idea that "it's good to stand in line for food" made recently by a politician still active today.

For example, there are two opposite interpretations of the injunction to "do unto others . . .," one of which involves doing kindnesses and the other of which involves getting back. Sadomasochists choose one or the other to have influence; sometimes (hypocritically) they choose to do both alternatively or simultaneously.

TO MAKE ONE'S SADOMASOCHISTIC INDIVIDUAL IDENTITY CLEAR TO OTHERS

Issues related to sadomasochism become a great part of "who I am," by implication reflecting on "who I want to be" and "what I should be like." For such individuals, "who I am" in terms of a carefully hewn self-identity proudly paraded is more important than being sincere and right about what is moral and acceptable. Their self-identity is often not so much a formed view of the ideal "me" as a way to remove themselves from the constraints of the outside world and live in an almost spiritual world of their own, where this identity involves a separation of themselves from everyday reality/behavior. Not surprisingly, they object to anyone trying to bring them back to ordinary worldliness, believing others to be insensitive/uncomprehending. For example, one individual I know has a number of active and lively, even believed to be alive, tutelaries in her life; she objects when her husband tries to force her back to skip the tutelaries and, realigning with reality, take care of her real children. Her identity is as a Shakespearean "Queen of the Fairies," as she actually seems to prefer living in a parallel universe that only a select favored few inhabit. She has no friends, but she does have a fairy ring made up of bushes transplanted around her home in a circle specifically arranged to attract frogs and other little creatures. Regular people she ignores as "not being of my sort."

DUE TO WANTING TO BE COMPETITIVE (AND WIN)

Sadomasochists see most other people, including themselves, as adversaries and try to put them down so that sadomasochists can beat what they believe to be the competition and be the ones on top. Oftentimes their dominations supposedly indicating strengths are compensations for what they believe to be their weaknesses, in particular their feeling helpless to change and thus to master certain of their forbidden urges—not a few of which they recognize as being potentially harmful or unlawful. Oedipally fixated, their adversarial needs often symbolize the desire to beat out one's father in some competition, generally involving fantasies of their own making, because losing a competition to dad, or to those who symbolize dad, is unacceptable simply because they are living out their need to best an uninterested father figure, literally if not figuratively whipping him in some sort of pitched battle of the minds that only exists in their minds.

In life, they feel disappointment and humiliation when compared to almost everybody else. Cruelty to oneself and others is their way to give them a leg up in this arena by getting there first with abuse of all concerned.

AS A WAY OF MASTERING TRAUMA

Masochism represents an active mastery over the potential for passively experienced trauma. Masochists unconsciously activate/orchestrate the repetition of childhood and even newish traumas to avoid being ambushed by the same or similar traumas once again along the lines of been there, done that. When trauma can't be avoided, it can be at least provoked on schedule at a time when one is more ready for it, or if not really ready for it, now still in a position to more effectively defang it should it occur seemingly spontaneously (as an ambush).

AS A WAY OF DEALING WITH LOSS

Represented too is fear of deprivation, for here one is awarding oneself as something special after not getting it from another person, perhaps forcing others to give it to them out of a sense of responsibility and/or pity over having been neglectful.

AS A WAY TO EXPRESS PHILOSOPHICAL PESSIMISM

As masochists, these are individuals trying to avoid the doom they feel to be inevitable in their lives. They are pessimistic individuals for whom feelings of the potential for extreme defeat to come prevail overall. Happiness can only be potentially fantasied and never fully achieved/maintained. That everything must go wrong in their lives is a given. It is a given that compromised (faulty) object relationships are the best that can be hoped for and that satisfaction cannot be sustained in any given relationship without the crackups that are ultimately inevitable if a relationship goes on too long. The conviction that something bad has happened/is happening/must happen is affirmed via not only the sadomasochistic idea that nothing bad can possibly be avoided but also the belief that one will be responsible for disaster and so "I will be blamed," so that like Sisyphus the sadomasochist will suffer, as joy is always pulled out from under her/him as it is just about to be grasped, and the sadomasochist must not keep climbing toward nirvana knowing that it can never be in fact attainable, because fate and sometimes God do not wish it to be. The masochistic motivation here is "Why bother, for things will go wrong anyway as my fate and comeuppance." The sadistic motivation here is "I will get back at you for making my life miserable by clearly pointing out what you did to me, show and tell."

With masochists and pessimistic individuals, to some extent, as for most everybody else, a fear covers a wish: the fear that all will not go well covers the wish for disaster to strike. Feelings of extreme defeat to come prevail. Even a simple order from the grocery store is going to get messed up. And if it doesn't, these individuals find a reason why it will go wrong, complaining, for example, that the checker left out an item that they forgot to order in the first place. If one worry doesn't materialize, they can always bring another one to life.

AS A WAY TO EXPRESS OMNIPOTENCE

Individuals who claim they possess special powers or abilities feel that they can have special effects on others. These individuals are therefore able to put others to all sorts of tests while themselves presumably being immune to the effects of stress and failure and able to get away with anything.

Such individuals will act superior to others who compete with them as if possessing special powers or abilities that allow them to dictate to others who think they can dictate to them.

AS A WAY TO SEE IF OTHERS WILL HELP WITHOUT HAVING BEEN FIRST ASKED (BEGGED) FOR ASSISTANCE

There is a wish that others will act spontaneously to protect one from harm (e.g., one acts out not only the scenario of being harmed by everybody but also the related fantasy that one is safe, for others will see the problem on their own and don't need prompting to be called in as saviors to put a stop to harmful behaviors in the making). Masochists are too often afraid to ask for help because of a fear they will be turned down. For many, help that they have to specifically request is no help at all but is rather unasked-for/unwanted interference with their daily lives.

Testing others sometimes represents a wish to have one's (self-punitive) needs met without having to actually ask for them to be gratified. The hope is that others will spontaneously divine what is wanted/needed and come forth "with the goods." Other related factors involve a wish to be loved unconditionally expressed via spontaneous (self-sacrificial) behavior on others' parts. An element of "keep loving me no matter how hard I try to drive you away" is often present.

Testing other people's limits can be a motivation. This is related to the wish to be loved unconditionally (e.g., "even though I behave in this incomprehensible and even disgusting way with you, I still expect you to love me and treat me right").

Many sadomasochists enjoy setting others up to see if they themselves are truly loved. Thus, a woman gives a man a beautiful complex dinner but only, however, as a prelude to making an impossible demand on him: to please remove his new landscaping, for it is blocking her view. He finds her behavior intolerable and continues on, doing so without prompting and thus failing her test.

There is also a wish to protect others from oneself, from doing harm to them by sewing the matter up by doing the very same harm to oneself first before others can get involved on the same level. A fear of criticism and punishment exists, prompting the masochistic individual to get there first and so in a controlled way, as a known quantity and quality, that is, without being ambushed and so to say "spare me for I have done to myself what you seem to be intending to do to me."

In short, while some masochistic behavior represents a wish to have one's self-punitive needs met without having to ask for them to be gratified, other such behavior involves a wish to be loved unconditionally and spontaneously and not necessarily as the outcome of begging and consequent responsive behavior on others' parts.

A fear of physical harm experienced passively may be reduced by harming oneself actively. (This defense is called identification with the aggressor.) But perversely, sometimes masochism is a prelude to making demands that one hopes will be rejected, anticipating that others will not go along but will in fact treat one in a nongifting way.

AS A WAY TO CONTROL ONE'S FEELINGS

Implied in sadomasochism is the need to always be in charge of one's feelings. A fear of becoming overwhelmed and fragmented by one's feelings can lead to a masochistic shutdown. Sadomasochists also test what others can tolerate and renounce certain demands upon others out of fear that they will be rejected or drive others away.

AS A WAY TO BE DEFENSIVELY ACTIVE RATHER THAN PASSIVE

A fear of physical harm prompts sadomasochists to actively harm themselves and others to avoid being ambushed passively. They reduce the fear that something might occur passively by living it out actively along similar or the same lines. A fear of physical harm and death is here actively conquered by anticipating it and forcing it. Here masochism involves the retaining of control by leading instead of by being led. A woman constantly proclaimed that she wanted to die and expected to in three months. Then she discovered that it was her pacemaker chest battery that was about to die, so she disbanded a large party she had invited many to so she could get into her car and go home to get her replacement battery before the old one's juice ran out.

Masochistic symptomatic behaviors such as cutting often represent an attempt to control one's feelings perhaps via a process of displacement from an emotional to a physical pain.

Fears that others won't tolerate one get tested, as they are simultaneously part of a test of the fear of losing self-control/control over others.

AS A WAY TO CONCENTRATE FEELINGS

A fear of becoming fragmented by being flooded by inner feelings out of control leads to concentrating one's feelings into one or a few actions only so that feelings might be more easily held to account in their boxed-in fashion.

AS A WAY TO PROVOKE OTHERS TO PAY ATTENTION

A special fear that masochists have is fear of emotional or bodily harm by sadists one has presumably provoked. Certain antisocial behaviors such as urinating in public belong here as symbolic of a need to startle others into paying attention and giving permission by ignoring what is happening. A significant wish to communicate one's needs to others and see who is paying attention is at times simultaneously present. Murder often represents among other things another person's fury about being treated badly via being ignored. Some murders can be prevented by not treating others who are on the edge in an unsympathetic or cruel fashion, hearing them out with sympathy rather than asking them to attempt to bottle themselves up out of consideration for others.

AS A WAY TO DEAL WITH ANXIETY

In exceptional cases sadomasochism can have tripartite-structure qualities just as any other psychological symptom. Many masochistic behaviors are anxiety/fear-driven: sadomasochists seek relief from an anxiety for which there are many reasons, mostly involving a panoply of forbidden wishes about to break through, inflaming conflicts between aggression and pity/succor. A compromise formation is sought, combined as a wish to hurt others and a fear of hurting them; as the expression goes, "You only hurt the one you love the most." Such a compromise formation is a way to express fear of hurting others and the wish to hurt them at one and the same time.

Sadomasochism is generally initiated by the superego, which causes the release of anxiety related to guilt (about being a bad person). The literature emphasizes how in sadomasochism guilt is often of an oedipal origin (e.g., related to unacceptable murderous/sexual feelings toward the parent of the same sex and rivalrous feeling toward the parent of the opposite sex). The misdeeds and "evil" thoughts in question on the others' part may be more imagined than real. There is less anxiety if wishes are controlled by prohibitions. One thinks, "I want to be me because, see, I am a good person for not gratifying my basest instincts."

The nature of the guilt is generally related to the nature of the imagined or actual personal misdeed(s), emanating from the id. It is here that various (sexual and aggressive) instincts lie, perhaps dormant but ready to break through with a specific stimulus from within or without.

However, masochists anticipate shaming and self-loathing even when they did nothing wrong or have even done something right so they can say, "Please don't attack me, can't you see that I am already someone who has been busy attacking myself?" or "Please appreciate what I am already going through." Interpersonal suffering sends the message, "if I am already down, then it is less likely that you will want to knock me out."

A savior complex may be a way to avoid anxiety. Here one is proud of oneself for giving something up, relinquishing to others what one oneself would want to have (and/or need). The belief that it is more blessed to give than to receive prevails in the masochist's armamentarium. (Sadomasochists don't fully explain why this self-sacrificial stance should be so common.) One prefers to make oneself saintlike, making oneself weep in order to self-sacrificially avoid making others cry. Self-sacrifice not only avoids anxiety; it also gives pleasure directly. Anxiety is also the product of failing to meet the dictates of one's ego ideal—the belief, or certainty, that nothing will ever go as expected or as desired based on one's fondest hopes and dreams and expectations of oneself and out of life. Anxiety can thus be reduced by lowering one's self-expectations.

A fear of submission/need to be dominant is an ideal that often characterizes the ego ideal of sadomasochists. According to some observers, there is an unconsciously driven triumph over those who try to help; this is in part due to an ideal of being independent, related to a fear of submission, or, paradoxically/conversely, a wish to submit to humiliating control. Hence the masochistic triumph that says, "You see you can't do anything for me no matter how hard you try. If I let you do anything, it would mean that I am weak."

However, once again, masochists anticipate/accept shaming and self-loathing even when they did nothing bad or have done something good so they can say, "Please don't attack me, can't you see that I am already busy attacking myself?" and "Please appreciate what I am already going through." Interpersonal suffering sends the message that if I am already down, then it is less likely that you will or will even want to knock me out.

For these individuals, success is perceived to be the equivalent of failure due to a success phobia and also due to the zero-sum fearful belief that anything I get, someone else will lose exactly, qualitatively and quantitatively. Subtle rationalizations come knocking here such as "My rivals wouldn't want me to succeed, and I am doing obeisance to them." For example, we hear from the individual afraid to be a winner how pleased he is as he says, "It's a shame; he is the same age as I am, but I am being so much less productive than he is" or saying that "It enhances one's morality if one has to wait in line for food."

Masochistic patients let abject altruism and empathic caring relieve their anxiety in full anticipation of knowing that "I am a good person who does unto others before I do for myself."

AS A WAY TO BE UNRELIABLE AND COVER IT UP

At times, sadomasochistic unreliability is their way to hurt family and friends and create real problems for other people. For example, a neighbor, already hated for constantly putting her garbage out as close to her neighbor's property line on her own large estate, offered this neighbor a tempting business proposition, only to subsequently change her mind about going into business with this person—after this person quit her steady job, leaving her as a victim floundering with no source of personal and financial support, ultimately to lose her house and have to move in with her mother just to be able to eat. Their word is unreliable, their promises are rarely kept, their signed contracts are rarely enforceable though they look good on paper, and in general these are the individuals who when they say "trust me" mean exactly the opposite and go on to act in an entirely untrustworthy mirror-image fashion. Hurting people as if they themselves were psychopaths, they feel very comfortable in those social areas of life where shady practices produce the best rewards and no demilitarized zone ever invented by man can function in a truly protective way for their potential victims. Narcissism gets into it too when their wish for success motivates them to the extent that they have very little concern for who gets hurt in the process.

They say they do such things as sign unenforceable contracts and enter into invalid agreements because these distract them from a constant feeling of boredom and emptiness that plagues them underneath it all.

But in fact, it is their narcissistic need for feeling justified for being oneself, for being who they are, that surpasses any concern they might have about how their victims will fare at their hands, and they even have the gall to come back to the scene a year later and suggest "let's not let hard feelings permanently ruin our relationship; let's try again to be friends and even give one another a shot at going into business together." In effect they have become psychopathic-like sadomasochists hurting others via turning on the charm. Some even resort to claiming illness to explain their misbehavior, and they become functionally good at this, putting one over on others again like the psychopaths they can be and whom they emulate, especially when cornered. Often they play the sick role, as they cite fearing closeness to isolate themselves from others. Finally, they tend to refuse to take responsibility for themselves, hurtfully blaming the other person for their failures in what are supposed to be joint missions meant to be the responsibility of two individuals right from the start. Now instead of condemning themselves as criminals, they condemn their victims for being suckers.

In the ambivalent mode, sadomasochists as children and later as adults are first seductive, then negative and rejecting, having a "go away, come back I love you" interaction whereby they ask for a positive relational response and then abandon others as soon as they get it. An expressed combined fear of hurting others that merely softens their true wish to hurt them is often present and characterizes the ambivalent relationships of those sadomasochists who proclaim to be object dependent as they manifest a clear wish not to ever be alone, only to get discovered cheating on their spouses.

There is a fear of being left alone that as a complaint provokes others to do just that: to leave them by themselves. Before suiciding, a 70-year-old person says, "I don't want to be 85, living by myself in a one-room apartment, never going out, having food delivered with nobody visiting me." All his friends abandoned him because they felt that he was complaining excessively about something that would be unlikely to happen in his case. The masochist's special fear of being left alone seems almost self-fulfilling. Any fear that this might actually occur arouses spite in those potentially poised to comply and leads to isolation or further isolation (e.g., fear about the possibility that one is in immediate danger of being or in the throes of actually being completely isolated). Prematurely concerned that others will mistreat them, masochists paradoxically deliberately provoke others to mistreat them in just the way they fear might happen, doing so just to say "I told you so" and "I am too smart to let this happen without seeing it coming."

A fear of being alone leads them to attempt to control the other person to get them to say "I will never leave you." But often their motivation is paradoxically to urge others to leave them. Their neediness soon becomes off-putting. I know of some people who send others an e-mail and then a few more in a few minutes if they haven't heard back just to reassure themselves that they are still in the other person's favor. This annoys others, and the overeagerness causes others to drop them precipitously.

AS A WAY TO TAKE ADVANTAGE OF OTHERS

An individual asks somebody if he can use his winter home for a few weeks and then when given permission to do so turns the heat down so low to save money that he freezes the pipes. While the homeowner is visiting to see how things are going, another guest arrives, and just to impress this guest, the first guest acts as if the house is his. The homeowner then turns the radio on to a station he likes; the guest turns that off and puts on another station that is the one he wants to hear. He doesn't follow the rules to not pick up people for sex but instead turns the place into a virtual haunt for deprived lovers so that other men's wives, as the neighbors say, are coming and going all day and night. Finally, when the owner needs some storage space he offers him one or two of the unused rooms, only to then ask the owner to remove his stuff since a friend of his, someone he really likes, will be moving in shortly. The relationship between sadomasochism and narcissism and selfishness becomes clear.

AS AN EXPRESSION OF THANATOS AND EROS

Thanatos struggles with Eros as both contribute to the final picture of sadomasochism. Manifestation of the death drive takes a number of forms. These may include destructive envy of others and ruined important opportunities for success and happiness in their lives leading to requests for pity, as they convince their therapists of the hopeless nature of their situation, though their need for pity in fact is the product of their own past behavior. (Pity involves hopefully corrective contrivances on others' parts; for example, they beg others to "help me and feel for me" instead of criticizing me for what I did to my life and giving me advice about making necessary changes.) Political expressions of Thanatos involve debates and rallies whereby one side's objective is to put the other side down without being at all cooperative or considerate and getting a job done. The rationalization is winning when in fact expressions of anger and rage at others contribute to most of the final problem.

Eros takes the form of making too many enmeshment demands on others, ultimately driving them away out of a need they have to self-protect from being overwhelmed.

AS A DISPLAY OF VIRTUOUSNESS

Self-defeating behaviors can exist side by side with areas where social and personal success rule—ones that are compatible with the patient having a good and productive lifestyle/relational history/work history in many other situations and not necessarily having an impossibly difficult lifestyle in all venues. It is as if these are two different realms, so the two should not be confused as if one can't be a good leader while having bad relationships with the women or men in one's life, even being a sexual harasser while retaining the capacity for being a genius in the realm of political savvy.

AS A WAY TO EXPRESS AGGRESSION/ANGER

Aggression is a major force in sadomasochistic symptom creation, yet the role played by aggression is ignored by too many experts trying to discover why people become sadomasochistic. Hence, we need to study and seek to explain the metabolism of aggression (which besides the sexual instinct is one of the basic instincts that form the basis of sadomasochism.)

Due to ambivalence, which consists of one part anger, sadomasochists are often unclear about what they want from other people, and they make that felt. In business, a boss angry at his or her workers sometimes prevails even when the anger interferes with the making of good business decisions.

The so-called masochistic fear of hurting others and the willingness to take it on the chin oneself to spare them is very often not the empathy and altruism it first resembles but instead is merely a roundabout way to hurt others along the lines of "see how you have made me suffer" and "now what are you going to do about it?" This seems to have been the case for the woman who presented herself to the world as an animal lover, only to herself commit suicide for very little reason, leaving all of her five dogs homeless and thus displaying the utmost of cruelty to that animal who was herself.

Sadomasochists unerringly focus in on disappointing people, setting the stage for them to be their victims by disappointing them and stirring up to greater heights the anger others already feel in their bones.

Aggression as a drive is often managed by moral sadomasochism (telling others "one just doesn't do that or feel that way"). At times it may be lived out interpersonally in one's sexual behaviors (e.g., whipping). When aggression is turned on oneself suicide may follow, an aggression to the self mainly meant for others in fantasy if not in action. (Hence the appropriate reaction to a suicide. As an internist speaking of a patient who committed suicide said, "I feel spooked." As another said, "I just can't stop missing her, Doc; what am I going to do to feel better?")

Some goals of aggression are to increase others' tension, to tweak another's superego as a punishing agency, or to bring another person down for not seeing the world as one sees it oneself. At times the sadist plays the role of a punitive conscience or is a stand-in for/representative of an omniscient society that supposedly always knows what is right and what is wrong and for all concerned, however hurtful it may be to the inhabitants of a certain culture. In a recent case a leader drove a strong business out of the community by his insistence on certain moral principles that not everyone shared. Manifestly preoccupied with making society a better place, he failed to notice that his personal onslaughts on the community made it an unfriendly place for acceptance of his principles.

Masochists often turn into sadists by offending those who love them, provoking them to withdraw their love, possibly for a good reason, from the other person and also possibly from themselves. Disappointment, expressed or not, is often provoked in people who right from the start have had such a high need for love that they become increasingly aggressive at the first signs of potential rejection, to the point that their objects feel helpless to know how to respond to what they feel to be the less than supportive input coming their way.

Alternatively, the masochist selects others to mistreat him or her or simply allows others to do so by failing to protest. Masochists fail to say "no" to mistreatment about to come or actually coming their way; rather, they say "yes" to potential mistreatment in the offing. They seem to welcome it; the fear seems to come with a wish—a fear of being mistreated coming with the wish to be abused. Sometimes these individuals put love to the test with provocation to see if the test will or will not be passed, and generally failure awaits. A woman tests her neighbors' patience by decorating a common hall in a way that she likes however much it offends everyone else, old dried flowers not being one of their things.

Patricia A. Cross and Kim Matheson note that psychological and physical hurts are variously involved. So often when given a choice of partners the masochist selects the most unsuitable one and regrets, not inappropriately, this selection all one's life. Pursuits of the unattainable and refusals to retain the desirable are commonly distinguished properties of such relationships. However, these authors "found no support for the view that sadomasochism as an illness . . . reflects sexual guilt on the part of masochists . . . or is an id-driven behavior [that] differentiate[s] sadists from others."[1]

AS A WAY TO REDUCE PRESSURE FROM THE SUPEREGO

Reasons for limiting oneself in terms of gaining pleasure are usually described exclusively as a phenomenon related to a need for self-punishment, which is in turn related to guilt, but they can be sequelae/complications of other motivations (e.g., of striving for more power than one can expect to handle/reasonably achieve). That is, sometimes they are not id but rather ego ideal driven.

Mostly if they sense the achievement of pleasure, the next issue that countervails is unconscious guilt, and this is often (but not always) over incestuous oedipal strivings. Pleasing or displeasing the poisonous introject becomes of primary importance, and this is diverting because pleasing or displeasing real external or internalized objects should be of much greater real-life importance to the sadomasochist.

Many observers note that in sadomasochism, we see dominance of severe superego pressures inducing guilt and inducing the need for self-punishment for the conscious/unconscious implication of sexual and/or aggressive impulses. Clinically, this is often dealt with by cutting, which reduces the intensity of intense affect and/or chronic tension. Here one lets off steam by "opening up the sluice gates," illustrating the literalness of some sadomasochistic activities and actions.

AS A WAY TO EXPRESS ENVY AND COMPETITIVENESS

Envy and competitiveness are core issues for these individuals. They can't tolerate being outdone by anyone. One way to deal with envy and competitiveness is by retreating into obscurity; another includes avoiding competitiveness by strengthening oneself so that others don't represent nearly as much of a threat—to outshine other people while cutting off their source of light, making these others feel helpless.

Sadomasochists, many of whom are fixated on the oedipal level specifically, where they compete lifelong with the parent of the opposite sex in terms of power and the search for glory, see most people, including themselves, as their adversaries and try to put others down so they can become even with or beat what they believe to be the competition. And it appears that everybody is the competition. Sometimes they dominate others to compensate for what they believe to be their own weaknesses, in particular their feeling helpless compared to some vaguely defined ideal. A child-man's need to best some father figure leads later in life to feeling disappointment and humiliation when compared to almost everybody. Others can be readily hurt by the sadomasochist's obvious and constant envy and active competitiveness.

AS A WAY TO MAKE ONE'S ANTIPLEASURE STANCE CLEAR TO ALL CONCERNED

Unconscious attachment to damaging, selfish, cruel, demanding, primary, usually severely narcissistic, objects persist from early childhood on, as the individual has become accustomed to at home being part of the scene where parents advocate for the unsuitability of certain gratifications, forcing one to be brought up in an atmosphere where certain pleasures are forbidden and the wonders of certain displeasures, such as absolute sobriety and other absolutes that are the antithesis of joyfulness, are strongly advocated. The parents who condemn family members in hushed tones for always having a cocktail every night before dinner so vociferously that the son or daughter can practically smell alcohol on every sinner's breath with each and every contact (disgusting sot!!!) teach the sadomasochist the regular critical words that come to mind with each and every contact with someone who looks to be a potential imbiber or epicurean on any level.

AS PART OF A CONSTANT NEED TO EXPERIENCE/FOSTER HURTFUL INTERPERSONAL FANTASIES

The mind of the sadomasochist is built of numerous layers of critical and unloving thoughts about oneself and others. This state of affairs is strongly maintained, for like sadomasochism itself on all fronts it makes one feel alive and connected. Exciting struggles between evil and good (evil winning) being desirable are retained without there ever being any resolution, although with shifting mood there may be a change in the balance.

AS PART OF A CONSTANT WISH TO RILE OTHERS UP

It is exciting for the sadomasochist to feel able to induce intense negative affective responses in another person. This he or she can accomplish by merging excessively with or being excessively remote from another. Many sadomasochists prefer to make life into an exercise of suffering for themselves and for others as well. If someone asks a reasonable question they might just not answer it, instead attacking the questioner for being mean of spirit or intrusive behaviorally.

Bullying

Bullying seems prevailingly sadistic, although one can argue that the ultimate consequences can be masochistic in those cases where the provocateur (such as the individual teenager doing the bullying) winds up getting stabbed or shot for being that bully. In such instances it almost seems that considering the expected retaliation to come, the bullying one is as much of a masochist as he or she is a sadist.

Case: I was very upset because of the conditions my son revealed that he has to work in (as an assistant clerk in the criminal court). His coworkers, it seems, have a grand old time making fun of him—grilling him as to "what he will be doing over the weekend" (e.g., are you going out with a girl?); telling him that his hair is thinning or frizzy or that he needs his bangs trimmed; and calling him either a MF'er or a PAB (punk ass bitch) "in jest" (reverse racism?). According to my son, who tries to laugh it off and just keep to doing his work so as to not make things worse, he even has to eat lunch alone in his hot car in the parking lot just so as to avoid the lunchroom. (One can ask here "Why does his car have to be hot, and shouldn't he be meeting the bullying head-on?" and answer these questions "because he feels as if the bullying is deserved, and he is treating himself in a way that accords with the outcome—he is self-defeating in accord with his desire for future abject self-defeat.") Masochists owe it to themselves to be future oriented (e.g., to anticipate how every act of their youth holds as a prospect for problems for the future); they should especially remind themselves that nothing they portray about themselves ever disappears from the Internet.

AS A WAY TO SHOW HELPLESSNESS AS A FORM OF MASTERY

Helplessness is a form of mastery used by sadomasochists. They cite the centrality of helplessness and the belief that the helplessness in relationship to inner and outer forces is a form of mastery leading defensively to its opposite: the controlling nature of (sadomasochistic) relationships formed. The helplessness here relates to one that infants quickly pick up that expressing pain (discomfort) gets mother's immediate attention.

There is an infantile omnipotent belief in the power of pain as it determines immediate and effective attachment to others; that is, "if I seem to hurt, and do hurt you, you will come to me." Even the toddler has an awareness of the power of angry thoughts and feelings and sees that normal assertiveness itself can be omnipotently destructive and therefore might sometimes ought to be restrained (e.g., via masochistic control in the form of self-defeat). In the omnipotence that is an aspect of helplessness, the individual responds to stressors by acting superior to others as if he or she possesses special powers or abilities and therefore is immune to the effects of stress and anxiety.

Paradoxically, then, complaints about relationships are designed to foster them.

AS PART OF MAINTAINING THE PARENTAL TRANSFERENCE RELATIONSHIP

When parents are not attuned to the child, the child becomes frustrated, then takes his or her frustration out on him or herself, it having no other place to go. The lack of attunement that is characteristic of such children's lives in turn leaves the child in the position of violating the rights of others, making masochism itself sadistic because the masochist is treating others in a way that is the antithesis of (healthy) attunement that the masochist lacks and wishes for.

Toddlers generalize (transference involves generalizing) the behavior of their own parents to all other adults, so that if their own parents react negatively to a certain type of behavior, the toddler believes that everyone else will too. This makes it hard for the child to credit his or her own later experience to the uniqueness of the experiences with his or her parents (e.g., for the child, it is as if other grownups are all just like his or her punitive parents). Thus, the child expects in his or her pursuit of the avoidance of misery, pain, and suffering that other people will react like his or her own parents did under similar circumstances. The pursuit of suffering then becomes a major organizing unconscious motivation characterized by the parentalization of all others.

Treatment involves cognitive separation individuation: correcting the idea that not all parents are the same, so one is predictably going to be treated shabbily by all others as one was treated by his or her own parents. It also involves self-organization: deciding who I am (e.g., a good person) and regulating one's own self-esteem accordingly, not just according to what the child thinks his or her parents, or their substitutes, likely think of him or her.

Some children are unable to see others as they really are and so cannot see how they themselves are treating others (often masochists themselves) in a way that is the antithesis of (the unhealthy) attunement that their parents had with them.

AS AN AFFIRMATION OF THE OVERARCHING INFLUENCE OF SELF-PSYCHOLOGY

Ornstein notes that in what is called "self-psychology," the origins of sadomasochism, as with other forms of personality disorders, can be traced to "*lived experiences* rather than to drive-related fantasies (e.g., of an oedipal nature) from the past."[2]

AS A WAY TO BE SPITEFUL

Case: Today was déjà vu with loving Sis; remember when she would not give me the name of her cement repair guy, even though she gave it to all of her girlfriends? Well today, she wouldn't give me the telephone number for my uncle who is in rehab after being in the hospital for 3 weeks—she has been calling him every day, but suddenly she "doesn't have" the number, or has to look when she gets back to her desk, or will send it to me when she gets home, then when she gets home she can't find it. OF COURSE SHE CALLED HIM ON HER CELL PHONE SO IT IS RIGHT ON HER DEVICE. I asked her why she is always so mean to me and what is it to her to give me his number. She said you can look it up. Then I called her a bitch—which she is, and she said "I'm going to tell EVERYONE you said that." What is she TWO YEARS OLD?

AS AN EXPRESSION OF GUILT

Guilt is an important stumbling block for sadomasochists, particularly but not exclusively for those who are primarily masochistic. When it comes to feeling guilty, sadomasochists are unlike borderlines. In the former case, sadomasochistic guilt is pervasive and constant, while borderline guilt is intermittent and unpredictable as to what elicited it in the first place and what caused it to peak/subside. In the sadomasochist, the guilt one feels is mainly not only constant but also fungible; that is, it applies to almost everything they respond to and do. But in borderlines, the guilt they feel is strongly confined to episodic, here-and-now aspects of things, particularly relationships.

Guilt forms intermittently, often depending on the stage of the relationship (merging, emerging, or in between) they are currently caught up in. In the one case, sadomasochism, guilt reins in patients, stopping them from certain actions of which they might subsequently disapprove; in the second case, borderline personality disorder, guilt being missing for long periods of time allows for certain atrocities (during the guilt-free period), and all sorts of unruly things can happen when in guilt-free periods these individuals feel unduly permissive toward themselves and others. (Only later, for reasons unfathomed, they can go into a serious rage with other people, leaving their victims to themselves feel guilty as well along the lines of wondering, "What did I do to deserve this?")

AS A WAY TO ADVANCE TRUTH AS PART OF A DEMAND FOR ACCEPTANCE

In their relationships, they use people to enhance pride and avoid its fall. They want to be seen as special and to be comforted and soothed as such. They want to appear as perfect, in the sense of being shamelessly good and powerful, and feel helpless if others don't view them that way. One patient bragged that the president of the United States visited her three times, landing his helicopter on the roof of the condo she lived in. Although it is documented that she did know him personally and had a large terrace, I think that her tale of the visits was an elaboration of reality.

AS A REFLECTION OF ONE'S STUBBORNNESS

There is a "see if you can stop me" calculation aspect of cutting and anorexia, as mentioned throughout. Others try and try but can't prevail and so can't stop the major and minor self-destructive mutilations, ranging from eating thumbtacks from the hospital bulletin board to other more minor masochistic interactions with a sadistic impact. They feel harnessed as if they are in the employ of another one holding the reins and others determining who is in charge. There is a fear of deprivation lest one might lose one's bragging rights and can no longer be the one proudly determining what is acceptable and what is not.

AS A WAY TO MAINTAIN THE CLOSENESS TO OBJECTS/HANG ON TO THEM

Sadomasochists don't see other individuals as either all good or all bad; rather, a synthesis is made to characterize the full relationship. For borderlines it is just the opposite. Others are generally evaluated steadily, that is, every day the same way. Sadomasochists' objects are more of stable than shifting proportions. Splitting, on the other hand, is characteristic of borderline relationships and encourages the instability of relationships so that borderlines generally have positive and negative relationships one after another, each with the same or a different person, perhaps going at one and the same time.

The defense of compromise formation permits simultaneous gratification and punishment for forbidden (often incestuous) wishes. This is most clearly seen in sadomasochistic sexuality, which is neither exclusively painful nor fully pleasurable but is often both.

AS ITSELF A PRIMARY MOTIVATING FORCE (DEFENSE)

Sadomasochists use a primary sadomasochism already in place defensively. Sadomasochistic *passive-aggression* is a sadistic way to provoke another to become agitated and hurt; sadomasochistic *reaction formation* (blamelessness) is a way to assume innocence and finger a victim, a protestation of one's innocence that involves allowing oneself in a roundabout way (with excessive apologies) to attack others and put the pressure on them to apologize in turn and so deflect guilt. Sadomasochistic *rationalization,* often driven by resentment, is a way to justify one's feelings and actions whereby the individual deals with stressors by devising reassuring, self-serving but questionable, incorrect, or beside-the-point explanations and justifications of his or her own behaviors (e.g., "to forgive is divine"). *Daydreaming* (as discussed below) is a way to distort reality in one's favor, often by attributing exaggeratedly positive qualities to oneself or others perhaps in a kind of dream state. *Devaluing oneself* is a way to disclaim responsibility ("It's in my genes, I can't help it"). *Acting out* involves bypassing thought in the sense of behaving in a way that seems automatic so that not much or not any attention is paid to what one is doing, bypassing guilt by viewing one's actions as "not me," that is, too thoughtless/automatic to be me. And *repression* occurs when the individual becomes unable to remember or to be cognitively aware of disturbing wishes, feelings, thoughts, or experiences.

A fear of hurting others leads to defensive hurting oneself instead, thus sparing others pain by putting all the pain on oneself. A fear of being dependent leads one to play the independent role with others. The masochist feels that "I depend on nobody; I only need myself."

The active seeking for pain, punishment, and suffering transforms experiences of helplessness into an active hostile defense against being rejected. It is true in a paradoxical way that you can't reject (effectively at least) someone who is seeking rejection or who has been already actively rejected him or herself.

Like most or all other individuals with a neurotic complexion, certain other defensive mechanisms prevail with sadomasochists, including turning around on the self, leading to depressive tendencies; grandiosity (bragging about one's attributes to defeat people who might want to put their own on display); a need to be admired for one's altruism; distracting others from one's flaws via performing charitable masochistic acts (e.g., a man infuriating his wife by using their inheritance to buy a piece of land and a back hoe, then giving both to the church after letting both sit idle for years); a fear of being inadequate, leading to hypercompensatory adequacy behaviors (e.g., always coming to visit with excessively expensive gifts); a fear of being independent, leading one to instead play the sick role; and a fear of being sick, leading to hyperhealthy behaviors taking the form of extremes of independence that can be hurtful to others should others want to be at all dependent on themselves.

Prevailing is a wish to drive others away, leading to the masochistic avoidance that resembles avoidant personality disorder. The cry now becomes "nobody loves me," which represents an active arrangement rather than a passive victimization (as they often see it). Paradoxically, self-reliance is a pride they take in themselves.

When they are children their childhood superego makes them feel terrible rather than helping them regulate themselves (e.g., their self-esteem), so that they don't have to (just) feel guilty and helpless but can instead change in important positive ways. Therapy involves helping parents help their children manage negative feelings about themselves and deal with self-esteem and impulses in ways that are less pathological and minimally self-destructive to their developing relationships.

As noted throughout, sadomasochists relinquish their objects reluctantly. A wish to always be near to a significant other exists for many masochists. Behind the wish is a fear of making a relational mistake that might cause them to lose love objects they want to retain. Some masochistic relationships are motivated/retained primarily by a fear of being alone, which gets into it as sustaining the relationship. Because a fear of hurting others often prevails over the wish to hurt them badly, instead of assessing the validity of a given relationship, sadomasochists act out based on their own self-interests, as the sadomasochist ignores certain problems just to keep a given relationship going as anxiety-free as possible. Their cry is "I hope you will still love me no matter what I do and say." Typically a wish to have others come in and rescue a failing relationship significantly asserts itself. There is a wish for others to spontaneously intervene and to voluntarily come to the rescue to protect one from harm by acting as mediators when relationships seem to be in trouble. Masochists sometimes suffer in isolation, but sometimes they instead call for help.

Most sadomasochists want to have their needs met without having to ask for that. They wish to be loved not only unconditionally but also spontaneously (e.g., to have someone intervene without their having to ask them to do so). They then cling not only to the original relationship but also, when that is in trouble, to others whom they believe could save it.

A fear of being alone can present itself as a fear of hurting others, leading to defensive hurting oneself instead, or they play or exaggerate the sick role lest the other person in the dyad gives up and, overwhelmed by their neediness, abandons the relationship and moves on to someone else, someone more healthily independent. Thus, fears of intimacy and closeness are paradoxically there too virtually in equal measure. This is manifest in certain avoidant sadomasochistic behaviors whereby the prevailing goal is the contradictory one: to antagonize others so that they go away, thus completely destroying the possibility for even the remnants of a strong, lasting relationship.

The result is an admixture of hate and love; too often the former prevails over the latter.

In a sense, masochism = bribery and as such is a test of other people's tolerance; the hope is that others will welcome and accept certain sadomasochistic feelings and offer forgiveness or at least some positive feedback. But there is also a fear/conviction that others will find them intolerable and then protest and dissolve the relationship.

However, when it becomes annoying, as it too readily does, masochism = sadism, which can be off-putting. Therefore, as a test of other people's relational tolerance, sadomasochists wish to determine if others will or won't accept one's feelings and behaviors. The hope is that others will welcome and accept certain unique sadomasochistic feelings and behaviors no matter what.

Overall, masochists' self-esteem rises and falls with the number and intensity of their relationships (e.g., the number of "likes" they can accumulate on the Internet). The need for developing self-esteem from securing a relationship with somebody, even a stranger, gratifies them sexually, and success here prevails over the fear of rejection and isolation, leading to a vulnerable anxious focus relieved by attempting to merge perhaps with one given person only. The masochist can try to hide his or her flaws for the purpose of avoiding object loss. Certain masochistic acts and attitudes such as whipping represent an attempt, ineffectual/paradoxical as it may be, to prove love and enhance tolerance under the most difficult of circumstances.

AS A WAY TO SEND RELATIONAL MESSAGES (DEFENSES)

Masochists rarely cavil about telling others how they are dealing with stress/anxiety. They send messages by the use of the following commonly found defense mechanisms.

Acting Out

In acting out, an individual deals with emotional conflicts/internal or external stressors by firing first and aiming next, thus acting blamelessly because he or she is manifestly acting without reflection or apparent care and thus without responsibility for the negative consequences of his or her thoughts and behaviors. Acting without troublesome reflection or apparent regard for negative consequences and then excusing one's behavior through rationalization is a hallmark of this aspect of sadomasochistic behavior.

Passive-Aggression

Passive-aggression is a high-level defense whereby the individual deals with stressors not by acting without reflection or apparent disregard for the consequences to oneself or others as the height of selfishness (which one would think is the opposite of self-punitive behavior) or by being self-destructive in specific ways but instead by instituting a facade of overt compliance and even nobility to serve as a patina over the forbidden objective of displaying cutting hostility. Here there is hidden resentment, which may show itself not in an active-aggressive manner but rather in indirectly sadistic ways that are, at least to the uninitiated, hard to identify but nevertheless are as equally devastating to the victim as are overt temper tantrums. The most familiar examples of passive-aggression are racism and sexism, with instances of hate being justified by the racist as being reality-based in their entirety (e.g., being of statistical significance). Glass ceilings are the height of passive-aggressive "invisible" sadistic restraints.

A colleague would correct all my manuscripts after they were published, with no offer of editing being given before publication was forthcoming. The corrective suggestions involved issues where absolute clarity was no longer at stake and only matters of fine discrimination were of any real concern. Classification of him as passive-aggressive and/or sadomasochistic was appropriate but to him unacceptable and just another example of my mistaken belief that he was being not helpful but instead hostile. (I am keeping you back not because of what you are but because of the bad job you do.)

Projection

Projection is a low-level defense commonly employed by passive-aggressive sadomasochists—to give sadomasochism a raison d'être and as a modus operandi to express their innate aggression without having to take personal responsibility for feeling/being aggressively sadistic. A jealous husband is one who wants to cheat on his wife, but instead of admitting that to himself he accuses her of wanting to cheat on him first: as a provocation.

Homophobia based on projection of one's own homoerotic sexual desires and designed to appear in public, so to speak, in the form of thoughtfully considered, not irrational, hostile queer bashing takes sadistic forms ranging among assuring professional defeat of gays and lesbians by making them subject to glass ceiling containment to hurting gays and lesbians physically via gay bashing, cutting them down to size not only figuratively but also literally, as well as by familiar forms of overt violence to gays and lesbians (not generally considered to be sadomasochistic because deserved but certainly so in the opinion of some and especially in the belief of the victims).

Paranoia is rife in the sadomasochism of today's politics in which someone is taken down for some imperfection in a way that parallels how paranoid patients utterly destroy others for saying or doing something of no real consequence, for example, believing it sexist for having failed to use gender-neutral terms to describe someone sensitive to the usage of such language. Spreading paranoia can turn a whole society into an adversarial group operating in like manner at one and the same time.

Repression

Repression accompanied by denial, such as of one's own homophobic tendencies, is a high-level defense that when accompanied by reaction formation ("I am not defective, I am the next wave of progressive sociocultural development") and displacement (e.g., from disgust with gay sex to disapproval of gay marriage) reflects how homophobia itself is a projective defense against one's own unacceptable homosexual impulses (e.g., "I am not queer, I hate queers"). Thus, the more one hurts a gay person, the less one sees oneself as being gay oneself.

In repression, the individual makes certain that he or she is unable to remember or to be cognitively aware of disturbing wishes, feelings, thoughts, or experiences and actual actions taken. One holds back needed information/awareness simultaneously from oneself and from others. Such sadomasochists feel special resentment over being thwarted by others. They also believe that they should be able to do whatever they want whenever they want to, including being able to strike out when they feel struck down (wronged). Yet at the same time, there is a pressing hidden wish for and hence appeal to a strong ally/mentor to step in and help them impose control over their own personal impulses and protect them from themselves, protect others from them, and prevent retaliative mistreatment by others. Repressed memories may fall into this category or may simply be false memories not ever having been repressed because nothing happened.

Sometimes that which is repressed returns as a recovered memory alit by the associative process (e.g., something that "reminds" the individual of something else). Such recovered memories are hard to pin down in terms of being verifiable; often they do, however, have a clear sadomasochistic basis to them, which is the reason why in some cases they are invariably in fact being recovered deliberately to be hurtful, spiteful, and vengeful.

Rationalization

In rationalization, the sadomasochistic individual deals with stressors by devising reassuring or self-serving but fundamentally incorrect explanations of his or her own or other's behaviors. An attack on the self or on another person is thus persuasively justified/warranted as seemingly rational: "Of course that would piss me off. Wouldn't you feel the same way?"

In some situations the line between a pass, sexual harassment, and rape is often a very thin one, a situation sometimes exploited by individuals who know they shouldn't do something but do it anyway in a self-defeating manner, then excuse their intentions in creative ways to make their actions look like mistakes or accidents, anything but intentional, and not something to be punished for.

Daydreaming (Video Games)

Excessive sadomasochistic daydreaming (fantasy) is a substitute for human relationships and more direct and effective action as well as a deflection from actual problem solving, creating the passivity that is part of some aspects of sadomasochism such as a reason to remain asexual within a relationship. The daydreaming sadomasochist is also one who becomes suddenly and inexplicably unavailable when needed, though you have done many things for him or her in the past. Compulsive sexuality paradoxically belongs here and has a hold on the self perhaps to the point of compulsive cruising and attending orgies not only in private but in public places as well. The risk of negative outcome is not taken into account, as if one's safety and reputation are not on the line, and one's actions may leave a dangerous personal and professional trail behind. The gay man who hovers around the men's room seeking sex is an example of the sadomasochist who disregards the outcomes of antisocial actions.

Omnipotence (Knowing It All)

In omnipotence, the individual responds to stressors by making it clear to others that one is possessed of special powers or abilities, so watch out. Little or no awareness of one's own particular deficits is taken into account along the lines of "don't mess with me; you are just asking for trouble."

One of the goals here is to convince one's victim to yield "because I am stronger and better than you for emotional and physically rational reasons." "I know best" is presented as a primary delusion (I know it is so because I know it is so) not in the sense of somebody who really knows it all because he or she is well trained and well educated or, making a joke about it, he or she lives in New York, but instead by somebody well on the way to developing a savior complex without any evidence that he or he has been or will be so anointed. A comparison with another (inferior) person is implied. In politics, really devastating accusations are made toward another and then seemingly excused as reality just because one starts the tirade with "I have no proof of this, but . . ."

Omnipotence may be fired by a feeling of resentment over being thwarted by others. Most sadomasochists believe that they should be able to do whatever they want whenever they want and can arbitrarily withhold what someone else wants and needs. Yet at the same time, there is a pressing hidden wish for and hence appeal to a strong mentor to step in and help them impose control over their own impulses. Arguments with experts in the field are common, internal, and protracted (e.g., over which politician is or is not insane) and go nowhere. They are meant not to define truth but instead to defeat a rival. In this regard I think of the long lectures I sometimes get about which person has what diagnosis coming out of the mouths of rank amateurs. Some book reviews on Amazon.com reveal a self-image at work taking the form of "I know it all. Training and experience count for nothing." Tirades against psychoanalysis come from the mouths of those who have never even spoken to a real trained psychoanalyst.

Devaluation

In devaluation, the individual becomes hurtful/deals with stressors by exaggeratingly attributing negative qualities to others, perhaps for some peccadillo that is neither wholly forgiven nor ever forgotten. Life searches emphasizing prior peccadilloes are undertaken on a regular basis particularly involving criticisms of such activities as improper sexual advances that amount to very little (e.g., pursed lips to display one's fondness, not necessarily erotic, for someone of the same or opposite sex). There is something unbalanced about complaints of sexual harassment made by a medical student in an intensive care unit surrounded by people who are trying to save dying patients' lives.

AS A MANIFESTATION OF NONATTUNEMENT TO OTHERS

In the history of many sadomasochists is either a lack of or excessive parental attunement. This not surprisingly carries over into the common role played by the unpredictability of relationships that are generally in the sadomasochist either hypotrophied (unattuned) or hypertrophied (excessively attuned).

Sadomasochistic attunement can involve the wish to effectuate not love but rather control and dominance of others, to make others do what they supposedly ought to be doing, and to be admired/accepted for the intensity and seriousness of their relationship capacity and wish to have and keep others involved relative to an intensity and seriousness of the masochists' beliefs/involvements, reminiscent of the intensity of their involvements with their parents when they themselves were children.

Sadomasochistic attunement is itself a way to wake the other member of a dyad up to the significance and importance of another person, sometimes in effect even by suicidality as a means to beg for and get attention.

Personal and ancestral (DNA) masochistic anlage are involved as a way to demand reparation not only for what the individual's parents did to or did not do for him or her when he or she was a young child but instead in a backward-looking transference to demand reparation for what previous generations did to the ancestors of all concerned, taking it out on present company of the same lineage for what your great-grandfather did to my great-grandfather. Now they believe they have an excuse (reason) for their low self-esteem and a reason to be cruel to others retaliatorily, for they see it is a simple matter of purposes of reparation. The banners of some activist groups are thus formed and waved when "enemies" come into their visual/emotional field, and the groups come to see these others as socially provocative and demand reparation, their favorite expression (as they scatter the herb around) being "Rosemary is for remembrance."

In severe cases, the adult sadomasochist becomes a raging hostile tyrant whose present behavior is fueled by various negative emotions that are supposedly residua from the past, with today's behavior a desired compensation for ur-negative feelings relighted by present-day other people. Masochists look to beat up on other persons the way they feel their ancestors have been similarly beaten up on.

Because of a feeling of resentment over having been/being thwarted by others, sadomasochists conveniently believe that they should be able to do whatever they want whenever they want without caring much about what others think or do in response. Derangement syndromes that have a considerable component of paranoid protest in them contain a considerable streak of this resentment about how "some bloodlines" have been treated in the past and are similarly being treated in the present by others who are henceforward made to feel unwelcome in their lives (and sadistically rejected along the lines of what is considered to be "appropriate vengeance").

AS A WAY OF DEALING WITH TRAUMA

Masochism represents an active mastery in the here and now over passively experienced trauma from the there and then or in the here and now. Masochists unconsciously orchestrate the repetition of childhood trauma to avoid being ambushed by the same or similar traumas once again. When a trauma can't be avoided, it can be at least anticipated and thus prepared for. In post-traumatic stress disorder (PTSD) forms of sadomasochism, flashbacks might occur many years after a veteran's capture and forced march or after a pet's death. An individual finds him or herself repeating in spite of him or herself a painful scenario in anticipation of producing a reaction that this time around can be mastered. There is self-pity in oneself combined with a plan to bring terror to others via repeated complaints of "look what happened to me." As a result, there exists a combined fear of torturing others and a wish to torture them mashed up into one single symptom, an amalgam of a wish for pity and a desire for revenge.

Masochists do many bad things to themselves. One bad thing involves allowing themselves to undergo repetitive thought processes ranging from obsessive-compulsive personality disorder repetitive thinking to PTSD whereby the individual can't clear his or her mind of reenactments. In covalent PTSD, repeating the painful scenario to excess is the essence of self-abuse. One eye is always kept open in anticipation of determining others' reaction as the flashbacks are told and retold in a way garnered to get pity and to involve and torture the heretofore uninvolved person.

Distressing repetitive feelings also lead to distracting oneself via distracting tendencies often of hypochondriacal complaints (the content of one form of masochistic PTSD).

PTSD symptoms look but are not always under someone's control, illustrating how sadomasochism is more like a disease than a voluntary attack on someone, oneself included. The demands that patients with PTSD make on others' patience illustrate the intent of the PTSD disorder itself.

AS A DEMAND FOR A WAY TO REDUCE ANXIETY/TENSION

There is mystery as to the essence of sadomasochism, expressed in part as to why anyone should long for pain as a source of comfort and cause discomfort to turn into attaining pleasure. For some people, experiencing even a modicum of pleasure is forbidden, and that would seem to be for any one of a number of reasons. The commonest explanation is that a sense of guilt forbids one to experience pleasure either at all or as such.

Is the essence of the sadomasochistic experience an inability to process pleasure that the sadomasochist can't handle as such because he or she actually experiences pleasure as an unwelcome source of tension and therefore secondarily as pain?

But Reich questions his own formulation—that the masochist does not experience pleasure appropriately but instead experiences pleasure as painful—as being only partly true. That is, he says that the masochist does not merely experience pleasure as unpleasure. Rather, the masochist strives for pleasure like anyone else. But what happens is that a disturbing mechanism comes into play and causes this striving to backfire. Failing, he or she experiences a pleasurable sensation as unpleasurable due to the *intensity* of the experience, for when that exposure exceeds a certain intensity/threshold the experience is felt to be abrasive, as if things, being too intense, are just not going too well. The tension is experienced as an arousal from a steady state that is comfortable due to the absence of *tension,* including the tension that is part and parcel of too much pleasure (having too much fun). What occurs is that the masochist suffers from an intolerance of any form of psychic movement, arousal from a calm state (a comfortable condition with predictable parameters), finding the experiencing of an overproduction of feelings/emotions troublesome. Thus, the masochist doesn't mistake pleasure for pain or turn pleasure into pain and can even experience a modicum of pleasure as long as it isn't quantitatively excessive, but what he or she cannot handle is intensity of this or any other sort, so he or she avoids what would be a buildup of joy or of any other strong feeling. Masochism, then, is in essence a phobic mechanism whereby many individuals avoid feeling because feeling overwhelms them, much as happens to a bridge phobic who cannot drive over bridges. Here the height is not the only thing that bothers them; it is also the rush overall that the height (being out there with no protection and coverage) entails, providing too much for them to comfortably tolerate. The proof here is that many bridge phobics panic as they experience tension as they get higher and higher on the bridge, but as soon as they reach the apogee and begin to descend the anxiety abates because the rising tension is no longer a factor.

The validity of this theory depends on the accuracy of the central hypothesis of the abrasive nature of departure from the steady state. The paradox here is that while some masochists are phobic of tension and require tension abatement, not all are, for many of them actually seek tension enhancement (the equivalent of pain enhancement), such as the enjoyment of horror movies or spinning, even losing, at the gambling wheel.

The sadomasochist also seeks to enhance another person's tension on a personal level. This gives the sadomasochist power over the other person in a dyadic relationship. Thus, a relationship is avoided or abandoned if it is going too well and becoming, in the vernacular, "too darn hot."

AS A SEEKING FOR POWER

Some studies suggest that seizing power and not the giving and receiving of pain are primarily at the core of sadomasochism. Many such power-seeking activities, both of a sexual and a nonsexual nature exist for the sadomasochist and do so in various domains. The mentally unstable potential dictator and the controlling, misogynistic husband are examples.

AS PART OF BLAMING OTHERS, NOT ONESELF (DISPLACING BLAME)

Ancestral experiences are cited as justification for present resentments and lead sadomasochists to feel justified in continuing to demand reparation not only for what their parents did to them when they were young children but even in some cases focusing on a backward-looking transference to what previous generations supposedly did to their present-day ancestor. They put forth the hypothesis that ancestral masochistic suffering is a reason (excuse) for latter-day sadistic resentment that supposedly entitles the (narcissistic) sadomasochist to be an exception to the rules of the primacy of the present-day justices/injustices, hoping to justify acting as they already wish to do so via the sadistic omnipotent belief that ancestral injustices give them the right and power to do whatever they want to do to control the lives of those presently around them, because these other people come from an unacceptable stock.

In many cases, the adult sadomasochist becomes a raging hostile tyrant whose behavior is fueled by various negative emotions, such as envy, that originate in a Jungian past, the collective unconscious, supposedly as compensation for feelings of helplessness, discomfort, and shame induced by one's inheritance. And so they wish to beat the father and his father, and on and on, as an extreme case of retrograde oedipal rivalry in perpetuity prompting the vengeance of the ages—a rationalization for many sadomasochistic behaviors indicating a wish to retaliate against and get revenge on all persons taking on however remote a transferential parental role. Hence, one cannot control one's internal or external environment because it is, in fact, in one's DNA.

AS AN EXPRESSED WISH TO CONTROL OTHERS

Matters of control insert themselves and too often do so to supervene at all stages in sadomasochistic interrelationships—in the developmental and latter-day eras. For example, a man wanted to bring a heavy end table down one story. He wanted to carry it down, but his mother-in-law would have none of that: she insisted that he use the elevator to instead protect the physical integrity of his back. They argued to the point that a vicious power struggle ensued. He acknowledged that her intentions were good but that he felt that being 30 years of age, he could make his own decisions in this matter; she felt that because she was right, he was entering into a power struggle with her and because of it might hurt himself, and she wanted to make certain that didn't happen, so she made it clear that it was a matter of reality, not misguided intentions. There was no one right way here, of course; the issue was not the one right way (nobody cared to even think of that) but rather "one's way" and who was going to have it.

One element in all or almost all sadomasochistic interactions is the element of who is doing what to whom—that is, the matter of who is in control—with matters that assert themselves with relative spontaneity/ease and are therefore expected to come up sooner or later in any prolonged sadomasochistic relationship. Generally speaking, each member of a dyad forsaking the ideal of equality is struggling to be on top. I once advised a friend whose cat bit one of her friends to report it immediately to the insurance company. She reminded me that she was an insurance agent and already knew what to do. I reminded her that I was a doctor and knew plenty about cat-bite insurance, at least from the patient's point of view.

However, masochists and sadists control others differently, the masochist indirectly by whining and complaining and the sadist behaving more directly, with threats. Thus, different metabolisms of aggression are present, and different of its metabolites need to be identified and dealt with for each person in his or her own special way.

The answer to the question of why one would have to beat out one's spouse is as mysterious as is the question of why sadomasochists can't handle pleasure. But at the least the mechanisms are clear: the masochist controls more indirectly, by whining or even malingering, and the sadist controls more directly, by commanding. In a desire to get immediate results involving another person, his or her commanding nature emerges forcefully and takes over, when it might be better to just stand back and let what is going to happen simply happen on its own.

In the sadomasochist, the wish to control and dominate others, who must do whatever the sadomasochist wants them to do, often not only fails to get results but also starts a pitched battle, and most relationships can't withstand much of this.

A wish to always be in control of everyone exists to soothe the fear of never being in control of anyone. The latter represents a fear of being powerless and helpless as well as the paradoxical fear of being independent and being lonely, without anyone around whom one can control. The "see if you can stop me" aspect of cutting and anorexia (others try and try but can't prevail to stop the self-destructive mutilations such as behavior involving not eating) are often masochistic motivations harnessed in the employ of one being the person in charge, holding the reins, with I, not you, determining what shall go on now and what shall happen next, thus allowing one to be able to do whatever one wants without defeat looming in the wings.

Sadomasochism involves a wish to control one's own feelings as well as those of others. In particular, sadomasochism often expresses a wish to get relief from, by not being responsible for, feeling guilty about most things. It works this way: "I hurt you the way you want to be hurt; therefore, since you asked for it, it's not my evil doing."

DISPLACEMENT OF BLAME

Sadomasochism almost always expresses a wish to function within oneself or with others by reducing personal guilt by blaming others for being provocative. A woman tells a close friend of many years that she can no longer see him because she is suffering from an alcohol withdrawal syndrome. (He knows, and she knows he knows, that she doesn't drink.) He complains about the suddenness of the interruption of the friendship when he did nothing to warrant this. She shoots back, "You are constantly overreacting, here as well as elsewhere." The aim of masochistic suffering here as elsewhere is to blamelessly control others by displacing the blame along the lines of "you started it" rather than to change the self by first admitting culpability and going on from there, perhaps to apologize when one finally realizes that one is clearly wrong. Rules of any sort (e.g., that one must conform to the laws of biology and physics and follow social conventions) are deliberately undermined/broken so that one's misbehavior/suffering can be seen as blameless, because it is not the person but rather the rules that are defective. Control over the feelings and actions of others is achieved, but the transition to maturity/adulthood is consequently blocked because the individual, caught up in emotional vengeance, wanting to make others suffer and remove their power, ultimately winds up making him or herself suffer just as much or more instead. Delilah cuts Samson's locks; Sampson effectively brings trouble down on *her* head.

Sadistic behaviors represented here involve a fear of deprivation along the lines of "if you won't volunteer to give it to me, then I will wrest it from you." A victim in a double bind literally as well as figuratively has his or her hands emotionally tied. In this regard, some sadomasochistic behaviors are warnings of what might happen (to self or others) if one doesn't comply to the marching orders that are being handed down and comply right now.

AS A WAY TO WIN IN POWER STRUGGLES

The desire to be in control exists to soothe the fear of not being in charge, representing a fear of being powerless and helpless as if one is no longer able to function on one's own, so that one is no longer able to predict what the next moves are. A favored trick of sadomasochists is to ask for advice, then complain when it is given that "you are trying to run my life for me." Being in charge of one's life is of great, protective importance to sadomasochists, and to some extent it would have to involve a degree of irrationality including that associated with hypocrisy along the lines of "do what I say, not what I do." Sadomasochists who believe this put others in a double bind of the sort whereby they give opposite commands to themselves and others, and only one command can be followed at any given time without ignoring the other one.

Too, controlling others is a way to control one's own emotions. One's being the boss is a defensive figurative and literal deflection from one's being flooded by one's emotions and considerations of the outside world. Sadomasochism involves not only controlling others but also a wish to control oneself, one's own feelings and thoughts.

AS A WAY OF DEALING WITH GUILT

Once again, sadomasochism often expresses a wish to get relief by controlling one's own guilt feelings. It works this way: "I hurt you the way you want to be hurt; therefore, since you asked for it, it's not my problem."

AS A WAY OF DEALING WITH LOSS

Represented too are a fear of deprivation, for here one is awarding oneself with something special after not getting it from another person.

AS A WAY TO MAINTAIN THE JOY OF BEING SOLITARY

A song written by Barber describes the virtues of being alone with his pet cat, Pandur.[3] Some masochists, far from needing relationships, maintain and even foster the joy of being solitary (e.g., lest creativity otherwise be corrupted and turned into a source of anxiety, frustration, and helpless rage). One's admirable cognitive insights are even used to attack, humiliate, and drive others away, a "useful" technique especially for sadists who are inclined to be self-critical in the first place.

Some of the more schizotypal masochists don't want and need relationships to a great extent. This subgroup of masochists at best allows and even prefers attachment to a brutal, abusive, and sadistic object as a form of removal, with removal accomplished by fusing aggression and love, creating a (compromise) outcome as they use negativity effectively to neutralize the positive feelings in this as in all their relationships.

AS A WAY TO DEAL WITH THE FEAR OF BEING AMBUSHED

A fear of physical harm prompts sadomasochists to harm themselves and others actively in anticipation of being hurt (ambushed) passively, along the lines of "getting there first." A fear of criticism and punishment exists, also prompting the masochistic individual to get there first and so in a controlled, known fashion in terms of quantity and quality, that is, without being surprised but instead to say, "Spare me, for I have already done to myself what you seem to be intending to do to me." A fear of physical harm experienced passively may be reduced by harming oneself along similar lines actively, an action that by being anticipated can thus be brought under control at least in this one aspect.

TESTING OTHERS

All masochistic behaviors are fear-driven. Included here are the fear of bodily harm by others—sadists whom one has presumably provoked. Antisocial behaviors such as urinating in public test which cultural fears have teeth in them, that is, who is going to do what about antisocial behavior.

There is also a wish to protect others from oneself by sewing the matter up by doing all the harm to oneself before the other person can get around to being harmful.

AS A WAY TO SET OTHERS UP

Many sadomasochists enjoy setting others up; thus, a woman gives a man a beautiful complex dinner only, however, to give it as a prelude to making an impossible demand on him: to please remove his new truck from its parking space because it is blocking her view.

AS A WAY TO TORTURE OTHERS VIA UNCERTAINTY

Being unable to act/be certain is the masochist's way to tortuously suspend cloture by leaving all concerned uncertain as to where everyone stands and what comes next.

Masochists can be both full of pity and pitiless at one and the same time. A combined desire to hurt and a fear of having hurt others coexists simultaneously or sequentially. A painful amalgam consisting of ambivalence along the lines of "I just don't know what to do" is a typical scenario whereby sadomasochists seek to leave us not knowing where we stand with them and so not knowing what to do next to please or even to deliberately displease them (if that is what they seem to want).

AS AN EXPRESSION OF ENVY

Envy and competitiveness are core issues for these individuals. They can't tolerate being outdone by anyone. One way to deal with envy and competitiveness is by retreating into obscurity; another includes not striving for that excellence you are potentially capable of achieving so that others will no longer have reason to be envious of you.

AS A CONSTANT NEED FOR EXCITEMENT (MIND WORKS ALL THE TIME)

The mind of the sadomasochist is constantly thinking of different ways to hurt oneself and others; it makes them feel alive and connected. Exciting struggles between evil and good (with evil winning) make them feel actively and irretrievably doomed, which many profess to prefer over feeling depressed, lonely, and neglected.

It is exciting for the sadomasochist to feel able to induce intense negative affective responses in another person (e.g., to make the other person feel guilty, weak, inferior, and defective). However, the sadomasochist must always maintain a balance consisting of overwhelming anxiety involving the disruption of togetherness and abject dependency on an object outside of the self accompanied by the comfort of merging.

AS A WAY TO SEEK THE REALIZATION OF THANATOS'S PUNITIVE BELIEFS

Often the individual is uncomfortably followed around by powerful persecutory parental figures of "no" who keep the child/adult from going astray and whose voices later in life continuously appear at the moment of truth to warn against successful achievement. The point seems to be making all lives into an exercise of suffering for the child and for the parents as well.

There is the death drive in operation, and manifestations of this death drive take many forms. One's death wishes extend to many other people in one's orbit. These may include envy of others, prompting action, or ruined important opportunities for success and happiness in their own lives, leading to requests for pity (e.g., as they convince their therapists of the hopeless nature of their situation), a characteristic of their relationships that involves their looking for someone to pity them (which they perceive as supportive).

AS A WAY TO RELIEVE PRESSURE FROM THE SUPEREGO

Reasons for limiting one's pleasure are usually described exclusively as a phenomenon related to a need for self-punishment that is in turn related to guilt, but they can be sequelae/complications of other motivations, particularly of striving for more power than one can handle/reasonably achieve. Here, pleasing or displeasing the poisonous introject becomes of primary importance and diverts the individual from self-fulfillment.

We see the dominance of conscience activity inducing guilt and in turn inducing the need for self-punishment, generally for the conscious/unconscious potential or actual discharge of sexual and/or aggressive impulses, past behaviors, and fantasies about the positive outcome of future planning. Clinically, this is often manifest in cutting, which reduces the intensity of intense affect and/or chronic tension. One lets off steam literally by opening up the sluice gates, in turn reducing, or at least seeming to reduce, the intensity of built-up affect and/or chronic tension.

AS A WAY TO ENHANCE ONE'S SELF-ESTEEM

Low Self-Esteem and One's Ego Ideal

Low/lowered self-esteem is a dismaying, self-denigrating, demoralizing self-evaluation characterized by a loss of the positive sense of self so that the self is viewed as valueless. Indeed, viewing oneself this way sets forth an attitude that forms a kernel of one's self-view or identity as "dumb and stupid," and then one behaves accordingly by either treating oneself (or others) shabbily or overcompensating by treating oneself exactly in the opposite way. The feeling that "I as an individual am too stupid to have done better" is there even though should one fail it is not because of what one did but instead because there were no other alternatives/doable approaches or ways out of a difficult situation, so that one in actuality did the best one could have done given the circumstances yet still extends self-abuse for not having succeeded.

When lack of self-forgiveness sways one's self-attitude, this so fixes it however unfair this may be; then one goes throughout life treating oneself dismally, doing this to oneself as if one is an emotional pauper and then blaming others simultaneously (and sadistically) for one's plight, so that inevitably all concerned are seen as blameworthy in a situation that has been set up to virtually guarantee a negative outcome in this test of one's mettle/self-worth, one where the outcome is preordained.

Warped/lowered self-expectations characteristic of the nature of one's ego ideal are central to and characteristic of the sadomasochist. The warped self-expectations that lead to sadomasochism in men and women and to the fall in self-esteem that accompanies the sadomasochistic *anschauung* (personal outlook) arise from several seemingly diametrically opposite sources. The first is a lack of approval from critical significant others, forming the basis of one's superego and hence of one's guilt and by extension one's self-esteem. The second is a depressing dissonance between "how great I ought to be and how great I have and can ever become." "How great I ought to be" consists especially of gender-specific socially formulated/inspired idealistic self-messages along with material from others' input. Such matters involving being independent and being the provider, not the one provided for, lead to ego ideal dissonance, which results when there is a split between lofty or lowly self-expectations and actual accomplishments, as unattainable (lowly and lofty) self-expectations create familiar plaints and accordingly self-punishment fantasies such as "Maybe I have set my sights so high that nothing I ever do can satisfy me completely, or maybe I have set my sights so low just to avoid being predictably disappointed." Careful adjustments need to be made, altering the unrealistic assumption that we as individuals should always be able to predict what we can accomplish in life and can plan ahead to guarantee that we will accomplish just that. Rarely do things work out in the way we anticipate they will, another reason for self-punishment. Among some good rules about how to determine what to expect is to consider risk-reward ratios. Then we as individuals can avoid going on to savage ourselves for not having done things right and avoid attacking ourselves for having failed in these respects, a source of cruel punishment felt to be deserved and lived out in sadomasochistic thought and behavior.

AS AN AFFIRMATION/EXPRESSION OF NARCISSISM (ONE'S OWN NEEDS, OR LIKE ME AS I AM OR ELSE)

Sadomasochism is a very self-oriented state. Sadomasochists want others to accept them as if they go along with their values. This has a narcissistic function, one that attempts to influence others to be like oneself. It is closely related to know-it-all omnipotence. Gentle suggestions along the lines of "identify with me" are sometimes the point, but at other times sadomasochists, especially those in a group, tend to be too forceful about how and why others should live and be like them. Some are effectively acting out aggressive fantasies of complete domination of others and refusing to give up until others follow their lead, sometimes unquestioningly.

As already suggested, looking for admiration is part of the sadomasochistic picture. The wish to be admired for one's suffering on the one hand and/or one's powerful and influential cruelty on the other hand makes their narcissism into a major component of their sadomasochism. Some sadomasochists are motivated to seem perfect; otherwise, they beat themselves up figuratively and literally. Hope for perfectionism causes many of these individual to suffer until they get things right and thereby avoid being ashamed of themselves and offending others. Such a goal is never fully achieved.

Sadomasochists have the expectation that other people can read their minds and will become angered in the absence of compliance. You are supposed to know what is expected of you and then act accordingly. Their award ceremony needs to be anticipated and take place flawlessly as envisioned lest fear drive the possibility that others who do or do not know what is expected of them do or don't fail to come forth with what is required from them.

While the more narcissistic masochist doesn't want and need relationships to the same extent as other sadomasochists, stickiness of relationships still exists for them, and this means that a goodly number of masochists needing relationships strive to form and maintain them along preconceived lines, allowing and even fostering attachment to a brutal, abusive, and sadistic object, with object removal (active or passive) always anticipated with dread. For some such sadomasochists, the state of not forming relationships at all is perceived to be better than having relationships and then breaking up. For others, fused love and aggression exists and is indefinitely acceptable.

Oral deprivation leads to later demandingness, anal control leads to later stubbornness, and phallic fixation on a submissive-dominant continuum leads to later competitiveness and refusal to accept compromise, three of the problems almost always found to some extent in the run-of-the-mill sadomasochistic narcissist. Therefore, in the sadomasochistic narcissist, deprivation, control, and competition are chief sadomasochistic preoccupations and are all potential sources of grief for everyone concerned.

Developmentally, *oral* narcissists are those individuals who were either undergratified as children and so go throughout life trying to make up for everything they lacked as toddlers or were overly gratified as children and so as grown men and women become what I call "Pollyanna sadomasochists": those who rage because they always expect to be as completely fulfilled as they once were as children and hence as adults respond catastrophically to minor deprivations, which they predictably view as major deprivations. As narcissists, they expect that things will always go well for them and that all tragic events will bypass them. They find themselves shocked, surprised, and disappointed when some circumstances, as inevitably happens in life, turn against them. As workers, they become hypersensitive to criticism and respond to a boss who assigns them a menial task by thinking, "He or she is calling me a menial person." They also tend to confound constructive with destructive criticism and come to feel that any suggestion about how they might do better amounts to a tongue lashing about their having done badly. They themselves become sadists who seek out victims who are masochists, who themselves come to feel guilty for much of what they have done wrong (and are looking for partners to interact with).

Anal narcissists are those men and women who always feel that they ought and deserve to be in control of every situation and everybody and who rage and self-punish masochistically when they lack this feeling of having been gratified realistically or just feel ungratified in fantasy. They view anything less than full control and dominance on their part as a complete loss of being in charge and so as painful submission to others. Some were physically abused as children. Now as adults they respond negatively to anything that involves a complete loss of mastery over their environment, as once again they feel like children being beaten. At work these individuals, unable to separate their work from themselves, their professional from their personal ego, typically become depressed after confounding being appropriately supervised with being unnecessarily and unreasonably straitjacketed, and they see all requests made of them as part of a plot on the part of the higher-ups to regiment them completely and quash them thoroughly. They then lash out and retaliate sadistically for wrongs that haven't actually been done to them and in ways they as victims refuse to subsequently disavow.

Phallic narcissists are intensely competitive individuals who devote their lives to being numero uno and standing out from all the rest. As a result, they become easily disappointed when they discover, as they invariably do, that they are only one face in the crowd (e.g., are "big nobodies"), that they compete with many others for the finite few rewards available in this world, and that they predictably clash with other people who also feel entitled to get something for themselves and especially with psychopaths who deal with their own fear that they can only have some of what they want by stealing all they can get (from vulnerable others). Such competitive narcissistic phallic sadomasochists, feeling that it always has to be all about them, become angry when others show any inclination to want to share their spotlight and get particularly depressed and become full of rage, which they take out on themselves, when they feel that others, even in some minor way, have hogged center stage, whose boards they have become convinced belong only to them.

Narcissistic individuals routinely ignore people who are good for them and instead stick with people who are bad for them, as they align themselves solely with flatterers who, by propping up their self-esteem as if this were the only thing that could possibly matter, can make them feel good and right because now they tell them they are like a force in the world. In contrast, they feel little attraction to simple virtuous people who might not idealize them aloud but instead love them quietly, in the right way, and for valid reasons.

Generally speaking, the self-indulgent demands of narcissistic sadomasochists are characterized by an infatuation with themselves carried over to become an infatuation with their emotions and their personal needs. They use their sadomasochism to arbitrarily gift themselves as being that person with traits that by reputation, fact, and deed enhance rather than detract from their overall functionality, giving them a strong, recognizable, admirable profile as "that special one," with their narcissistic love having been installed as a way to improve their self-esteem by thinking that they are and act better (more independent, more powerful) than everyone else. Too, they devalue others to avoid being devalued by others, getting there first with criticism and rejection of others to thwart or reduce the impact of others' potential criticism and/or rejection of them.

There is a demand to be admired for the intensity, seriousness, and appropriateness of one's position and of one's purpose, however much that involves punishing/demeaning others. There may be a demand to be admired for being stolid in one's views and being unwilling to change them extensively, except perhaps to gain approval and maintain a shaky relationship by enhancing another's admiration of them. Some days it can be most unwise to get involved in political discussions with them.

There is a need to effectively communicate the specificity of their own needs to others for agreement so as to have others under their thumb, figuratively in relationships and sometimes literally in the sexual aspects of that relationship. Proselytizing, a feature of narcissism, has a narcissistic function, one that attempts to influence the other to be like oneself. It is closely related to know-it-all omnipotence. Here, gentle suggestions along the lines of "identify with and so be like me" are sometimes the point, but at other times sadomasochists tend to be too forceful about how and why others should be/live like them. In some cases, they are effectively acting out aggressive fantasies of complete domination of others and refusing to give up until others follow their lead, sometimes humbly.

12

Comorbid Contributions

By comorbidity, I mean that a disorder such as sadomasochism is part of another naturally affiliated disorder resulting in the formation of a mixed disorder, such as the (depressive) narcissistic-masochistic character described by Cooper.[1] In some cases primary sadomasochism is a vehicle for the presence and expression of symptoms of other disorders, as most or all sadomasochistic displays have elements in them that delineate other neuroses and psychoses. And in some cases other primary disorders turn out to have sadomasochistic characteristics associated with them. In turn, all psychological disorders are sadomasochistic at least in one sense: due to their tendency to be associated with and cause suffering and pain in others as well as in oneself, suffering being an integral part of the structure of all neuroses and psychoses. There are differences, however, between outcomes depending on the disparate ways the mental illness complex brings suffering about and the whys and wherefores of the suffering that turns out to be sadomasochistic.

Here are some examples of the admixture of disorders and the consequences of such admixtures. These are just a few examples of how all psychoneuroses and psychoses are vehicles for the suffering of the self-defeatist and/or making others suffer. For example, there is considerable overlap between sadomasochism (hurtfulness of others), paranoia (blaming others), and psychopathy (taking advantage of others). Among the complexes commonly associated with sadomasochism that contribute to the suffering associated with sadomasochism in the troubled individual and make trouble for his or her victim(s) are undifferentiated psychotic masochism, schizophrenic masochism, schizotypal masochism, bipolar masochism, paranoid personality disorder masochism, obsessive-compulsive personality disorder (OCPD) masochism, avoidant personality disorder (AVPD) masochism, histrionic masochism, depressive masochism, and passive-aggressive masochism. While all psychoneuroses and psychoses are vehicles for suffering, each makes the self and others suffer in different, often specifically distinguishable, ways. Thus, histrionic = panic in all concerned; OCPD = unremitting torture; schizophrenia = derealization (not knowing who, what, and where one is, almost always involving others in the dissociative process and sometimes eventuating in violence); bipolar depression = sadness for all concerned and manic high = excessive excitement, whereby patients are insufficiently calm but then are speeded up as their mind races and they become overwhelming; paranoia = suspiciousness; passive-dependent = feeling and fearing loss excessively and for little or no reason; AVPD = rejecting of closeness; and borderline = alternately devouring (merging) then regurgitating (emerging) objects in one's orbit.

Thus, many depressives disparage themselves in masochistic fashion, and many masochists disparage themselves in depressive fashion, in both cases turning this disparaging self-devaluing into devaluing others along ways similar to how they devalue themselves. This often occurs via the process of projective identification whereby one sees oneself in others and treats others similarly (badly). (In this chapter I discuss the admixture rather than try to discern which comes first and prevails, an insoluble chicken-or-egg problem.)

DEPRESSION AND SADOMASOCHISM

Sadomasochism is often associated with *depression,* as similar overall gratifications, inhibiting forces, and problematic object relationships (especially difficulties with dominant, critical others leading to excessive hurtfulness) are found in both.

Depressive low self-esteem is self-defeating: masochistic insofar as the self is the object of the low self-opinion and sadistic insofar as others are the targets of the defeating words and actions (projective identification) of the depressive sadomasochist ("I could have done much better than you"). In both, the blaming is assaultive and rancorous with the goal to produce pain, often in retaliation for some overt or covert insult, imagined or real.

Sadomasochism is also often associated with depression, because overall gratification, inhibition, and problematic object relationship difficulties with dominant or submissive others are found in both. Many depressives disparage themselves in sadomasochistic fashion and turn this disparaging devaluing onto others. There is a ready sharing of sadomasochistic/depressive pain along the lines of "I want you to know how I feel, and how you make me feel, and to make you feel the same way, even if it takes my being as cruel to you as I am to myself."

Provocation of another is central to the depressive (and often paranoid) process. The individual (subject) becomes keenly aware of how the other person feels and "where to stick the knife in." Moral issues are generally emphasized, making depressive sadomasochism a variety of moral masochism. In a self-sustaining virtually circular process involving escalating guilt, those of a depressive nature goad a man or woman to actively have, accept, welcome, and elaborate guilty feelings and then to act them out self-destructively, thereby becoming even guiltier in retrospect about having acted stupidly punitive.

"Should-a" and "could-a" are prominent aspects of the sadomasochistic loops that get formed and become preoccupying. They may originate within the individual or be started up by another person eager to form a pathological dyad and refusing to let up.

In accepting depression and its ravages as expected (a part of life) and then rationalizing the depressed state as good (or at the very least not so bad because, for example, it heightens sensitivity) and so not doing anything about it, such men and women remain passive in the face of their depression after convincing themselves that they are simply beset by misfortune and that fate has abandoned them temporarily/permanently. They see their failures in life as not due to depression but, rationalizing things, as instead due to circumstances and bad luck that they 'cannot now or ever have changed / controlled.'

Acceptance or even enjoyment of defeat is common. As previously mentioned, if such a man or woman is depressed about having a bad job, he/she even convinces him/herself that this is a good thing because the most painful jobs are the best jobs in the sense that they are the ones that come with the most job security or benefit society the most.

In enjoying depression as if it is such sweet sorrow, some depressive sadomasochists even have or develop an addiction to depression whereby depression becomes for them a singular way of adaptation, a friendly habitat, that is, a welcome (habitual) venue of thinking, feeling, and behaving in a mode not to be gotten rid of but instead to be clung to enjoyably like one's best friend in a cruel, friendless world. For such men and women, what seems to others to be inordinate self-deprivation and lack of self-indulgence becomes a preferred way of feeling and living and indeed, for the depressed sadomasochist, the source of some of life's greatest pleasures.

By not getting enough treatment or using what treatment they get as the way to keep their illness and with it their depressive suffering, individuals such as this favor the masochistic triumph whereby they say to themselves and to others, including their therapists, "See, you can't help me, for try as you might, I am destined to forever be sick, and so I am fated to always be depressed." This form of guilt comes so naturally to those who suffer from it that we are tempted to say that certain aspects of guilt are temperamental in the sense that they are inborn or native, more primary than earned/developed.

In hurting themselves mentally and physically, depressive sadomasochists may slowly commit suicide by drinking to excess, taking harmful drugs, injuring themselves at sports, purposefully having hurtful auto accidents, or exposing themselves to severe illnesses such as HIV. Or they may actually humiliate themselves physically or by adopting a hair shirt morality and acting as if everybody should learn about the wonders of wearing the thing. The depressed woman who slashes her wrists or cuts her body or develops a suicidal anorexia nervosa to self-punitively waste down to nothing has as her counterpart the depressed man who has a sex-change operation not to be true to his inner self (perhaps the more common and rational motivation) but more so to self-punitively have an excuse to mutilate his genitals precisely to devalue what he has been given by God and what he already has, is, and does with it.

Depressive sadomasochists relate mainly or only to others who treat them shabbily. They find and form the closest relationships possible with society's major guilt inducers. They deliberately seek out and try to enlist the approval of people who are negative to them, trying their hardest to get those who formerly openly disparaged them to change their minds, come around, and think otherwise, the typical sadomasochistic mission to convince one's worst enemy to become one's best friend. Such a man might actively take on romantic challenges that are the most difficult or impossible to meet. Such a woman might seek out all the wrong places to look for love.

Though they seek solace, they are nevertheless lonely because they refuse to compromise in their choice of who they love along the lines of "for me, only the very best will do." Though they themselves are not entirely prize-worthy, they continue to look for the perfect mate and find too many others unsuitable. Paradoxically, they also passively accept without protest whatever victimization comes (or they can bring) their way, because this offers them the satisfaction of knowing that they are in fact being brutalized in exactly the same way they feel they deserve and ought to be.

They won't accept good advice along these (or any other) lines precisely because it might be helpful to them in the short/long run.

In developing creative or writer's cramp whereby instead of getting openly depressed they deliberately work below par or do some specific mechanical damage to themselves, they become like (according to legend) Robert Schumann, who may have deliberately damaged his fourth finger by using a device of his own invention that in fact hurt his hand and deprived him of aspects of his career as a concert pianist.

Many depressed sadomasochists are sadistic, as their sadism arises out of an unfortunate but prepossessing metabolism of guilt. Masochistic depressed men and women mainly punish themselves; sadistic depressed men and women mainly punish others. A patient was once the principal of a school; he turned in a bunch of students for using pot, and they threatened his life. Henceforth he punished himself by refusing to leave the house lest he be attacked and hurt by the gang he turned in. One Christmas a depressed woman, who refused to recognize that her son was schizophrenic, reacted to his being 10 minutes late, though he promised to show up on time and was looking forward to a beautifully prepared meal, as if he never came at all, even though this was the only time he was 10 minutes late, and cut him out of the will in retaliation for his unsupportable behavior.

Depressive low self-esteem is unabashedly self-defeatingly masochistic insofar as the self is the object of the attack of low self-opinion and unabashedly sadistic insofar as others are the target of the blaming of an assaultive nature with depressive rancor (e.g., over how you mistreated me [brought me down]), amounting to a reason in both instances for the ready sharing of depressive pain. Life searches in which the individual goes back over and over his or her life trying to reedit it, dwelling on all the mistakes he made in the past, are descriptively and psychodynamically both depressive and sadomasochistic. Depressives such as this fail to accept the fact that they couldn't foresee the future and so blame themselves as if they screwed up deliberately by doing such things as choosing a profession that unforeseeably turned out to be unpopular and not remunerative.

Many depressives disparage themselves in sadomasochistic fashion and turn this disparaging devaluing onto others, then retroflex it back again on themselves, blaming themselves for what they feel they did wrong.

In short, depressive low self-esteem is masochistic and vice versa insofar as the self is the object of the low self-opinion and sadistic insofar as others are the target of blaming of an assaultive nature, with interpersonal rancor central to the causality in each case.

There is a ready sharing of sadomasochistic/depressive pain/attack with one person in a dyad or group at a time or with many simultaneously. Not everyone, however, is treated equally simultaneously. Some are set apart to be immediate targets of the blue mood, while others are spared for a time or a lifetime until circumstances change and new reasons appear to attack. Love objects become hate objects virtually overnight or after a long positive relationship has developed and lasted, seemingly forever. In some cases the victim doesn't see it coming; in other cases there is a long sadomasochistic evolution consisting of "how I don't want to be your friend any longer," triggered in some instances by the most trivial of circumstances. In one case a man called his friend to tell her that the restaurant they were about to meet in was a cold place, so bring a sweater; this she misinterpreted as an attempt at controlling her and ended the relationship on that account alone. Events of a trivial nature that occur within families, especially between parents and children, often set off relationship-ending interactions.

Sadomasochistic men and women remain passive in the face of their depression by convincing themselves that they are simply beset by misfortune and that fate has abandoned them permanently, and, rationalizing their failure as not due to depression/themselves but to circumstances, they blame their nasty fate on bad luck, convincing themselves that they did nothing to bring it on, and so there is nothing they can ever do to change things. For these reasons, many depressives actually accept feeling depressed and are reluctant to put forth the effort to change things because "why bother, it's inevitable." Besides, depression hurts, so we should expect a masochist to appreciate that and want more and more of it.

When antidepressants don't work, it may be because the individual is fighting them; antidepressants begin to work, but the patient doesn't like feeling normothymic (normal and not depressed) and resists their antidepressive effect in part because if not depressed he or she now no longer has any reason to complain as much as before. In enjoying depression some men and women even seem to have an addiction to it whereby depression becomes a singular way of adaptation; it has become in effect an old friend, a desirable habitual thinking, a feeling and behaving mode not to be gotten rid of but instead to be clung to enjoyably like one's best companion in a cruel, friendless, disappointing world. For such men and women what seems to others to be inordinate self-deprivation and lack of deserved self-indulgence becomes a preferred way of feeling and living and indeed the source of some of life's greatest pleasures. Secondary gain prevails; all the perks of being sick come into play, and in some instances it is even a pleasure to have someone else dress one and tie up one's shoelaces because this, however unneeded, still becomes an unarguable sign of being loved and cared for, so why give it up. The status of "poor, needy me" prevails, and the implied control over others assumes major proportions.

In not getting or using treatment as their way to keep their illness and with it their depressive suffering and their need to continue to cause others to suffer, men and women such as this when in therapy often favor the masochistic triumph whereby they say to themselves and to others, including their therapists, "See, you can't help me, for, try as you might, I am destined to always be sick, and so I am fated to always be depressed." In such cases good advice is ignored to the point that meaningful interpretations that might help anyone else are pooh-poohed, as is support from others in the form of "I see you as a better person than you see yourself."

These men and women often willingly substitute impaired pathological object relationships for healthy interactions with people. The most sadistic thing one person can do to another is to break up suddenly, without any apparent reason and without giving notice. In such a case the victim gets depressed, taking sometimes weeks or months to get over it if he or she ever does. Often enough there is no warning, and the other person doesn't know what hit him or her. Now the victim gets especially depressed not only because of the loss factor but also because of the seeming inability to foolishly have anticipated the nature of the event. The sadist is aware of what he or she has done, which is one reason he or she did it this way in the first place—a form of hurtful unpredictability, one of the favored tools in the sadist's armamentarium. Some are aware of how to make others feel depressed and go to it with great gusto because it largely satisfies their sadistic impulses, doing so all the more because of the hate implied. A lover gets up in the middle of the night and says, walking out the door, "I am leaving you" (and going back to my old lover). The victim never forgets this.

Excessive Altruism

Some sadomasochistic men and women behave in an excessively self-oriented narcissistic fashion. For example, they collar people and unload their problems on them, hogging the conversation and showing little or no concern for anyone but themselves. At a family dinner they look at their reflection in the silverware over and over again to admire themselves or make certain that nothing is amiss that might make them appear to be inferior to others.

Underneath, however, some are just the opposite of narcissistic. They are excessively empathic and altruistic individuals much too concerned about others' feelings to the detriment of their own. Such individuals fail to be adequately self-protective and self-gratifying and give too much to others while taking too little for themselves, even giving family heirlooms away as a statement that they no longer feel they belong. The narcissistic element in altruism is often apparent however much those who are altruistic hope to hide it in this way (beneath its opposite).

PASSIVE-AGGRESSION AND SADOMASOCHISM

Like sadomasochists, passive-aggressives want to keep a relationship going even though it is marred by an excess of hostility.

Passive-aggression is by nature sadistic to others, with the indirect aggression even more sadistic (due to being illusory, along the lines of "you can't prove that I am angry with you") than direct aggression. In each case the aggression is turned upon the self to become self-defeating. But in altruism where being kind to others is in part being mean to oneself, in passive-aggression being mean to others is in a roundabout way a method of being kinder to oneself. Here, being mean to others is disguised as being kind to others (e.g., inappropriately fooling oneself that one is being nice/kindly by hiding an attack upon others in the form of what at first appears to be an innocent question, such as "Just curious, unlike last time, did you vote the same way this time around?").

OBSESSIVE-COMPULSIVE DISORDER AND SADOMASOCHISM

The obsessive-compulsive symptom generally contains as both its goal and its predictable effect a form of self-torture or torture of others in an involvement that others likely find difficult to escape from due to the intensity and pervasiveness of the emotional enmeshment (some will tolerate this for the sake of the relationship overall). Obsessive-compulsive disorder/OCPD sadistic individuals, depending on their particular style, can effectively torture others with their worries and concerns. A father continually asked his son to "time me a minute" so that he could check his own heart rate and make certain he hadn't had a heart attack; alternately, he would constantly ask his son to find him the tape measure (he wouldn't spend—that is, waste—the money on more than one) so he could measure his legs to determine if he was suffering from a neuromuscular wasting disease. He was both masochistic in the sense of his constant worrying and sadistic in the effect he wanted to produce on his son: a kind of reverse Oedipus that had as its intent massive attacks on the son, thereby disabling him as being effective competition for the mother's love.

Some hoarders belong in this category (e.g., the woman who saved half of all her birthday cakes and piled them up in the living room, to the great consternation of the rest of the family who lived in the house and wanted the room for other, better things). Too often with hoarders we see the saving part when what is actually pleasurable is the spending part; here the hoarder is being sadistic by wasting the household money on junk.

NARCISSISTIC PERSONALITY DISORDER AND SADOMASOCHISM

Cooper has argued that the narcissistic function of characterological masochism is so inseparable from the self-defeating behaviors that characterize sadomasochism and identify sadomasochistic personality disorder that the concept of "narcissistic-masochistic character" is warranted.[2]

Some sadomasochistic individuals are openly selfish and narcissistic. Some instead display their selfishness and narcissism as its opposite: by seeming to be excessively unselfish and excessively hopelessly altruistic, only they are this way to the point that they allow damage of others and self-damage to occur. Their concern, self-concern and concern for others, comes across as an attack on others. These people look but are not just the opposite of narcissistic. They seem to be simultaneously excessively empathic and altruistic individuals concerned about others' feeling to the detriment of their own. They seem to be adequately self-protective and self-gratifying and give too much to others while taking too little for themselves. They seem to deprive themselves of what they need and long for even to the point of giving away their most treasured possessions (a possible warning of a suicidal attempt in the making). Here it is their invasiveness, not its content, that flies the sadomasochistic banner. They are making themselves central to a relationship perhaps in a way that makes them less desirable than they are proposing to be.

There is a controlling message in both narcissism and sadomasochism, for in both we hear "I am, but you are not, the legitimate boss in this relationship."

Narcissistic issues of adult life go back to early narcissistic injury, leading to later self-image distortions and self-esteem (regulation) concerns as a consequence of the disrupted caregiver-child relationship. Narcissists reject their children by being too self-concerned and hence bossy to let the child contribute much. At the same time, many are too thin-skinned to the point of walking away from a relationship at the slightest provocation they feel doesn't suit them. Responses to even the mildest rejection by others are often stereotypical and characterized by an "understandable" wish to retaliate and to get revenge on these others for being hurtful. Prevailing is the wish for being admired as special, associated with predominant underlying feelings of entitlement and omnipotence that, when disrespected, leave the sadomasochistic narcissistic person feeling treated like dirt, almost figuratively.

Later in life, narcissism consists of a symbolic reactive response whereby being hurtful to others and oneself exists in reaction to the feeling that one is inadequately appreciated and supported. We often hear "You can't treat me this way" when in fact the treatment referred to is the essence of ordinary (and that may be the problem). One asks a reasonable question, only to hear in reply "How dare you accuse me of doing that."

Characteristic too of narcissists is their expectation that you can read their minds and/or should know already what they are thinking without their having to explain themselves.

There is a close relationship between sadomasochism and narcissism in the sense that both affect the personality by permanently interfering with the development of a consistent and stable self-representation of a fully adequate person. Early traumas that disregard/wound the reasonableness and sanctity of the self have a significant effect initially and later in life are typically reopened and repeated in an attempt to master them ("this time things will come out all right"), because while they may lie fallow in interim periods of time, they have often become ingrained in the personality and are ready to be revived under the right circumstances.

Narcissism and masochism are inextricably bound together. For example, these individuals' "extraordinary suffering" "entitles" them to special recognition and to be an exception to the rules, so that they feel entitled and paradoxically feel self-loathing ("not entitled") at one and the same time. This has sociological implications as well for hate speech in which such individuals condemn others (or groups of others) for not having suffered as they have and go about making others suffer in retaliatory fashion.

They like to see what they can get away with to the point that they at times resemble psychopaths playing dangerous games. One dangerous game is that of "social justice" whereby people who were formerly hurt come out fairly ahead, while those who formerly hurt them find themselves this time coming out behind. This focuses on the victim and away from the victimizer.

Hurt feelings associated with being rejected by others are often characterized by a wish to retaliate and to get revenge on these others ("How dare *you* treat *me* with such disrespect!"). Thus prevailing is the wish to be admired as special, associated with persistent predominant underlying feelings of childhood entitlement and omnipotence that "must be respected in me as someone who is grown up now." Narcissistic preoccupation with the self leads to sensitivity about how you are treating me and rage if you treat me badly as well as lowered self-esteem if others seem not to appreciate how good and special I am, plus rage at those who don't see the narcissistic individual as especially entitled to being both outstandingly valuable (and yet as highly vulnerable as he or she actually is, or at least is perceived to be).

Often such individuals get into and remain in punishing relationships. They seem to gravitate to being taken advantage of, being abused, or having their positive contribution to a relationship minimized. Gone unrecognized is their own contribution to relational difficulties overlooked to the point that feeling unappreciated, they break the relationship up sadomasochistically (even when they and others feel and are needy).

Many have suppressed or otherwise made themselves unaware of others' angry disdain to the point that they continue to seduce people who ignore them rather than appropriately abandoning those who aggress against them. They are blinded by feelings of narcissistic entitlement that include an absolute inability to see why not everybody loves them.

Conflicts about attaining sexual pleasure prevail due to guilt, especially guilt in women about women being at all sexual in the first place, so that they remain in punishing asexual relationships because others seem to think that "women are too status oriented to want to have sex." Thus, women react by gravitating to being taken advantage of, being abused, or having their contributions and its magnificence go unrecognized as punishment for what they believe to be forbidden eroticism.

The individual who deals with stressors by attributing exaggeratedly negative qualities to self and others may seek a sense of being valuable through the identification with others. They have many friends and lovers hoping that this "golden circle" they surround themselves with will make them feel and look better to the world.

In summary, the partnership between masochism, sadism, and narcissism is relatively common, and the individual manifestations can alternate and defend against each other. The basic issue is who is giving whom support and positive feedback and who is getting pleasure by not being hurt. The masochist thinks about him or herself constantly from the point of view of the level of suffering of the self, whereas the sadist thinks about him or herself constantly from the point of view of "how much pleasure am I getting from causing others pain?," and the narcissist thinks about him or herself from the point of view of "to what extent being me is good enough for others to not mistreat me the way so many people do."

Sadomasochists and narcissists often act in similar or the same ways, though the motivation is different. For example, a narcissist gets a post office box in an inconvenient area just to be able to impress his neighbors with how his business is thriving, for they see him coming and going mailing and picking up mail. A sadomasochist, however, gets a post office box in the same inconvenient area, but now to be able to make it more difficult for him to keep up with his correspondence and easier for the neighbors to know how unsuccessful he happens to be (since he has to walk such great distances to pick up his mail).

There is a message of control in both narcissism and sadomasochism, with both along the lines of "I am, or am not, the legitimate boss in this relationship." A woman with agoraphobia so severe that she can't leave the house under any circumstances gets a post office box so she can tell her daughter "go pick up the mail for me, would you, please?"

Many seem to feel duty bound to their belief that there is something wrong with enjoying life and being happy in a relationship. Many, however narcissistic they may be because they expect so much, still feel guilty or anxious when experiencing positive feelings toward themselves and expectations of others.

AVPD AND SADOMASOCHISM

Many sadomasochistic individuals seem to suffer from AVPD symptoms. Here they feel duty bound to their belief that there is something wrong with enjoying life and being happy in relationships as much as elsewhere. Among these are sadomasochists who feel guilty or anxious when experiencing positive feelings toward others—positive feelings toward people that can even include themselves. (Patients with AVPD fear others and having relationships with them.) Some patients with sadomasochism even condemn relationships of all sorts and believe that it's better to be alone than to get involved with other persons.

Unlike narcissists, sadomasochists with AVPD may sadomasochistically remain in punishing relationships because these provide them with the distance they crave. They seem to gravitate to being taken advantage of or abused or to others who don't contribute their part to a relationship; only ultimately feeling unappreciated, they break the relationship up themselves or provoke others to do it for them.

Many such individuals remaining unaware even of the legitimacy of their own interpersonal needs have become too self-sacrificial to the point that later they come to resent what they have given up. Yet they continue to self-sacrifice and become increasingly isolated.

Many have suppressed or otherwise made themselves unaware of others' angry disdain toward them to the point that they continue to try to seduce people who ignore them rather than appropriately abandoning those who aggress against them—in this way assuring themselves that nothing will come from a certain relationship.

Conflicts about attaining sexual pleasure prevail due to guilt, especially guilt about being a woman who has sexual feelings in the first place so that AVPD women remain in punishing relationships because they seem to gravitate self-protectively to being taken advantage of, abused, or having their contributions and their magnificence go unrecognized by others who act as if they are unattractive. Many seem to feel duty bound to their belief that there is something wrong with enjoying life and being happy sexually. Many feel guilty or anxious when experiencing positive feelings of all sorts toward themselves and others. Negative feelings separate them from the feelings of closeness that cause them to be afraid and condemn others who offer them a hand.

When conflicts about attaining sexual pleasure prevail due to guilt, especially guilt about a man/woman being sexual at all, these individuals remain in punishing relationships because there the sex is forbidden/absent. As a consequence, the individual with AVPD is often a lonely isolated person or, if not, is one who forms relationships with others, only to abandon them in midstream on some pretext that is little more than a rationalization of the anxiety that promotes distancing in action. Those who are natively personally charming/appealing can do a great deal of damage to others who decide to become fond of them, leaving these others depressed and otherwise lost, unaware as to what happened to them—what they did wrong to provoke their own abandonment and whether they should try to themselves change to make things right again or just give up on the relationship.

Many AVPD sadomasochists convince themselves that they have what it takes to win a certain known AVPD isolate over; it almost never works, and almost always they come to blame themselves for having said or done something wrong to ruin a relationship.

Avoidant groups advocate isolationism as they try to attract people who want to share their distancing, even to the extent that they are without friends completely. Some are by nature inwardly oriented, giving them a schizoid flare.

In patients with both sadomasochism and AVPD, the individuals may sadomasochistically willingly remain in a punishing relationship as if they seem to gravitate to being taken advantage of, abused, or having their positive contribution to the relationship go unnoticed. Gone unrecognized is that their contribution is overlooked to the point that feeling unappreciated and guilty, they themselves break the relationship up masochistically and/or sadistically and even remain isolated or set out to find someone better.

Many such individuals, remaining unaware even of their own needs, become too self-sacrificial to the point that later they resent what they have given up for someone else.

Many men disapprove of women having sexual needs. They feel horrified about their wives or girlfriends being sexual and doing sexual things and hope/demand that they remain in punishing asexual relationships to make certain that women (as women = mother) aren't yielding themselves up to the sexual pleasure forbidden to women. Women who seek sexual pleasure are excused for doing so but are also accused of being taken advantage of, abused, or having their contributions and their magnificence criticized (the man's virginity complex). We sometimes even hear the word "whore" flung at them.

HISTRIONIC PERSONALITY DISORDER AND SADOMASOCHISM

Patients with a histrionic personality disorder and sadomasochism exaggerate the importance of humdrum day-to-day events, especially as these individuals overreact to real but minor slights from others and other negative behaviors on others' parts, in the vernacular making a big deal out of little to nothing. They also blow up the significance of positive aspects of relationships, especially those where physical closeness/sexual conduct is involved, often leading to false accusations of harassment and perhaps especially sexual harassment, although other venues are often cited, such as false recall of being set back unfairly in competitive relationships (e.g., "the election was stolen from me"). Since false recovered memories of seduction/rape can occur and may even be accompanied by the visual hallucinations commonly found in hysteria, such sadomasochists may develop the belief that others, who are in fact innocent, are trying to seduce them/have done so. The belief that someone groped them when it is not in fact true can be particularly hurtful/dangerous to innocent parties.

BIPOLAR DISORDER AND SADOMASOCHISM

Patients with bipolar disorder and sadomasochism display alternating elevated and depressed mood. Each mood swing is heavy on the hostility, especially in the sense of being intrusively hypercritical of oneself and others. They are easily confused with individuals who are paranoid, with at least one important difference: to a great extent they want and like to involve others in their moods as well as or more so than in their thoughts. This is in turn in contrast to those who are schizotypal/actually schizophrenic, who don't so much actively invite others into their affectively distorted and cognitively disrupted worlds but rather ignore those around them instead and treat them impersonally.

CYCLOTHYMIC PERSONALITY DISORDER AND SADOMASOCHISM

The role of anger is generally downgraded when discussing the mood disorders, of which cyclothymia is one. In this disorder, mood shifts are considered to be milder than they are in full-blown bipolar disorder. Still, the effects of mood disorders and sadomasochism combined, as with bipolar disorder, include despair and hopelessness. Cyclothymic sadomasochists can be very hurtful, as we hear the complaint "Boy, does he have a mouth on him." Once at dinner I just mentioned the name of a leader of men suffering from cyclothymia, only to have everyone else at the table, all of whom it is true knew each other, respond in chorus with exactly the same words and exactly the same expression: "everybody hates him."

SCHIZOTYPAL PERSONALITY DISORDER AND SADOMASOCHISM

Patients with schizotypal personality disorder and sadomasochism are suspicious, often paranoid, feeling that they are victims of mysterious forces from other worlds. In general, they experience all interpersonal relatedness as something problematic (*DSM-5*)[3] enough to stay away from other people who might want to get close. A certain strangeness pervades their whole being. Some other people like them that way; for example, they find otherworldly processes fascinating and enjoy entering with them, if only for now, into the spirit world of tutelaries and a range of other beings from the other side. Otherwise, their victims see their strange preoccupations as an attack on their own personal sense of reality and stay away in the belief that by getting involved they are blurring the line that should run between what is real and true and what is imaginary, however alluringly fairy tale–like the otherworldly events may be. It takes a certain kind of person to not feel put upon by schizotypal individuals and to enjoy the relief they give from considerations of the mundane world.

SCHIZOPHRENIA AND SADOMASOCHISM

The key to schizophrenia is its strangeness/bizarreness. There is a tendency to have false persecutory beliefs, and the patient's ability to strike fear into others' breasts over the possibility that they as troubled patients can become physically hurtful and do so without warning.

Some patients with both schizophrenia and sadomasochism tend to be extremely hostile, especially when it involves persecutory beliefs. All realms of hostile misbehavior consisting of hostility to the self and others are potentially part of this disorder. The individual who sucker punches a complete stranger on the street is likely to be on the schizophrenic spectrum and be acting out of a paranoid delusion about this other person, often about something that for anyone else would be trivial, such as "I didn't like the way his hat was tipped forward and he stared at me." Much of the world's violence today is the product of the behavior of those with schizophrenia responding to voices (command hallucinations). The absence of any social mechanism for forced treatment of people who are potentially violent (e.g., overseeing that those with schizophrenia take their medicine) is tragic, for these sadomasochistic individuals put not only other individuals but also society as a whole in a considerable degree of danger; yet depriving selective patients of their civil rights to freedom reflects poorly on all others in the world of schizophrenics, most of whom are not violent, making it difficult to institute effective measures of control on a general epidemiological basis. Additionally, psychiatry tends to shy away from identifying such individuals as violent out of the fear that they will be condemning all people who are mentally ill and especially paranoid schizophrenics, the vast majority of whom present no danger whatsoever to other individuals or to society as a whole, as being violent and as being worthy of being socially ostracized just for having one or more pathognomonic symptoms of schizophrenia. This makes it difficult to offer all patients the care they need and to offer society the protection it calls for at one and the same time. (Not taking their medication is part of their being hostile too. Our response consisting of not knowing just what to do for them is characteristic of that provoked by sadomasochists of all genres.)

Many of these individuals make up the homeless population. Our response to them, that "they are severely incapacitated," suggests that many of those we call homeless should instead be called schizophrenic, as some of these elicit a response in the general population that is not so different from the response elicited by others we call sadomasochistic. Not properly diagnosing a patient out of a misplaced need to avoid being condemnatory of innocents all over the world is a risky proposition when it comes to protecting the rest of the population. The use of diagnostic euphemisms (such as "akinetic mutism" for patients with catatonic schizophrenia) is charitable and kind to those who suffer from such a disease. But it is dangerous to populations at large because it doesn't point a way to treatment of the sufferer. Populations who complain that the individuals who silt up the best neighborhoods in town complain without recognizing that this behavior is not a coincidental by-product of their illness but rather part of it. (It is their sadomasochistic intention to do just that. Discussions about gun control after shoot-ups do not often get at the root of the problem. There is nothing more sadomasochistic in my opinion than walking into church and shooting at and killing large numbers of the supplicants.)

BORDERLINE PERSONALITY DISORDER AND SADOMASOCHISM

Patients who suffer from both borderline personality disorder and sadomasochism alternately devour and abandon others, in effect swallowing them up in the merger phase and then regurgitating them when disaffection takes over. Others are rarely aware of what they did to provoke the negative (borderline) behavior (and often in fact they did nothing, making the rejection, which comes eventually from all borderlines, that much more hurtful).

In the merging phase, some borderlines become emotionally enslaved to others, with varying effect on how others feel about that, while in the emerging phase the same borderlines will devalue and abandon others, sometimes these same others, with the almost predictable effect that others feel rejected by them without knowing what happened or why it occurred.

Hatefulness on the borderline's side is generally part of the picture rarely accurately identified, because much of the literature overlooks how hatefulness and thus sadism is an integral part of and explanation for borderline (and much other related) behavior. As with schizophrenia, the fear is that calling the borderline individual relationally destructive will be perceived not as a clinical evaluation based on careful, accurate psychodynamic observation of the effects that sadomasochism plays in having a negative effect on large populations but instead as a criticism, a pejorative comment about who this sadomasochistic borderline person is and how hateful he or she can be toward the victims with whom he or she comes into contact.

This we do know. In some cases, cutting seems to involve a split as the one person becomes two: the abuser and the one being abused.

PASSIVE-DEPENDENT PERSONALITY DISORDER AND SADOMASOCHISM

Patients who suffer from both passive-dependent personality disorder and sadomasochism often cling in such a way that others find them annoyingly intrusive, sometimes to the point that others feel beyond uncomfortable to feeling almost literally devoured. Others feel as if they need and want their space; the passive-dependent, however, wants to share their space too and has no intention of giving that right to others up. In a relationship they shadow the other person, hanging out with him or her when he or she gets dressed in the morning to go to work, even supervising his or her daily schedule by frequently calling to "see how things are going" and "where are you now?" Even simple stories about rejection cause passive-dependent sadomasochists to feel anxiety. One member of a dyad went shopping, only thinking that his partner was just taking a nap he chose not to leave a 'Back in 15 Minutes' note, throwing his partner into a real panic because he woke up alone and couldn't find a note telling him where his partner had gone. Passive-dependents often have little to no resiliency in this way: they figuratively put other people on a leash and leave it there, collar, identification tags, and all.

AGGRESSIVE SADISTIC PERSONALITY

In subsections of some societies, in occupational, political, interpersonal, and socioeconomic venues, patients routinely manifest Leary's "aggressive sadistic personality."[4] In these societies, aggressive sadistic personality seems to be the norm and can be diagnostically recognized not only by its own manifestations but also by the reaction it provokes in others. Even in social groups devoted to protest, masochism is often manifest from the start by the recognition of the inevitability of being punished (e.g., carted off to jail by the police), and sadism is often reflected from the start in the sadistic permissiveness involved in refusing to criticize/punish an individual for his or her clearly manifest indiscretions, encouraging by not discouraging them. The severe hostility between groups with different philosophies can be astounding and attributable not only to a personality disorder but also to a problem with temperament that these individuals feel they cannot control, and often they are right about that.

Yet because in some societies Leary's term "aggressive sadistic personality" covers many of these patients dynamically and descriptively, aggressiveness and sadomasochism combined seems to be too much the norm, which makes it questionable as a description of an abnormality (personality disorder). Some political groups feel that this is not a problem that needs to be cured but instead is a solution, a nirvana that needs to be maintained for specific positive purposes.

PARANOIA AND SADOMASOCHISM

Patients with paranoid personality disorder and sadomasochism are prone to making false and hateful accusations about others, stopping short, however, of having full-blown delusions about them. For example, false accusations of rape are sometimes as much of an aggressive nature (a way to make trouble) as they are of a sexual nature. (The accusations may be taken figuratively, not literally, or the other way around.) In general, false accusations about what others are doing to harm the individual abound (in both directions), are intended as agendas for typical sadomasochistic response to the sadomasochism, and often lead to hurtful accusations in both directions, the familiar circular firing squad. When delusions are present they often run deep, and these individuals can readily shift to becoming out of control and as such become somewhat or absolutely dangerous.

Paranoia is often confounded with bipolar disorder, since paranoid delusions of grandiosity can make the patient look somewhat euphoric/high (manic). But with paranoia there is no real joy, only attack contaminated by a joyless hyperactivity that has a different quality or feel to it than does true euphoria.

Diagnostically, paranoia and sadomasochism seriously overlap when there are paranoid vendettas, which may be against oneself or involve others. Here the suffering is attained through the creation of imaginary painful scenarios of attacking others/being attacked by others as supposedly rational reasons for attacking others/attacking others back. These are advanced along the lines of who did what to whom first, which generally involves the feeling that "I am attacking you back (for having wronged me)." The headline of sadomasochistic paranoid personality disorder might be one that refers to "who is to blame" (whether rightly or wrongly), really meaning who started it, and they, after assigning responsibility, go for the revenge in a fully preoccupied way that is as hurtful as possible.

Sadomasochists do differ from paranoids in one special way: the sense that paranoids get little to no true pleasure from their tormenting others. Their tormenting of others is not primarily satisfying but is instead essentially retaliatory. In a way, it is primarily defensive. These patients torment others to avoid tormenting themselves or as a way to get revenge on others for others supposedly having tormented them, as if others deserve being hurt and abused. Paranoia that looks purely like an attack on others is thus essentially self-protective in addition to being a simple release of anger. Sadomasochistic paranoids torment others not only because they enjoy doing so but also as a defense: as a way to avoid tormenting themselves or as a way to get revenge on others for others supposedly having tormented them, so that therefore being tormented is what others deserve.

Paranoid tormenting can be defensive, a first strike. The first step involves the displacement (projection) of blame along the lines of "I am not hurtful; in essence, I am just hurting you back in retaliation for something (however imaginary) you did to me."

Paranoid sadomasochists do also personally feel that they are tormenting others not only because this is what others deserve but also because this is what I and my victims/others would actually like (enjoy). One is dealing with the displacement (projection) of blame along the lines of "I am not hurtful; I am just giving you what you asked for (hurting you back)," the difference between pure pleasure and revenge (e.g., "my empathy and altruism lead me to understand and give you not only what you deserve but also what you might like").

Thus, these sadomasochists sincerely feel that they are tormenting others because this is what others want and deserve and because this is what others and themselves would like (enjoy) to have come their way. The second step involves "I am not hurting you, in essence I am being kind; you just want to be hurt (projection via empathy and altruism), so I am giving you what you want."

Furthermore, pure sadomasochists are rarely if ever voices-driven, whereas paranoids sometimes have command hallucinations; that is, voices are telling them to act as they do.

Hallucinations are rarely recognized as the full drivers of paranoid sadomasochism, but they are often part of the paranoid illness. The person who sucker punches or stabs a complete stranger on the street is often responding to voices and therefore is less "merely sadomasochistic" than suffering from paranoid schizophrenia. The man who cut up Picasso's *Guernica* likely thought of many things, including the harm he might have been doing to a society whose behavior he no longer wished to condone so that in a way he became part of the warlike depictions in the picture.

As with all paranoid vendettas, they may be against oneself or involve others or both, so that sadomasochism and paranoia overlap considerably. For example, suffering is attained through the creation of imaginary pain-filled scenarios of attacking/being attacked accompanied by supposedly rational reasons for feeling this way. The "commonsense response" is seen not as paranoia but instead as acting in a social way in an antisocial society.

13

Cognitive Causality and Therapy

The belief systems of sadomasochistic patients suggest a cognitive approach to understanding and treating some of their sadomasochistic problems. Routinely, subtle self-defeating cognitions creep into their functionality and lead them astray without their being entirely aware of what is happening and why. They reason their way into suffering and don't recognize it when they are marooned there.

These belief systems often overlap, and in the main are all derived from different forms of guilty thinking. Therefore, sadomasochistic thought and behavior is profitably viewed as the realization of the guilty thoughts one has throughout life from childhood on. Guilty thoughts (which in turn produce the pain and suffering of sadomasochism) are generally about punishment for forbidden sexual desires as well as various related and unrelated aggressions. Many of the latter are aspects of oedipal aggression. Thus, self-punishment is installed partly to mollify or avoid the perception or actualization of the danger of vengeance, personal damage, and hurtful abandonment likely as a consequence of long-term habits of inappropriate and appropriate competing in triangular relationships. The neutral ego, or self, needs to be punished, and the overly involved sadistic superego needs to do the punishing. In the masochist, failure and transgression are emphasized and brought up repeatedly as the driving force of one's identity ("I am a big nobody"). Resultant overwhelming emotional forces lead to fears of injury on the part of those others who in the first place seem to be the ones who have made one feel guilty or otherwise have done them harm. In short, an excessive unconscious sense of guilt creates pain that is payment for both past and present permission for current and further transgressions.

But this does not mean that cognitive therapy is the solution to all problems that sadomasochistic patients present with. Many speak of a downside that frequently plagues cognitive therapy due to its being dependent on cognitive logical correction. Helping all concerned (individuals and all members of a sadomasochistic dyad, triad, or social group) to become less unduly guilt ridden, depressed, and even suicidal and think more realistically and positively is an admirable and achievable goal. But underneath, such individuals are often hyperreactive people who are far too critical of, unsupportive of, or even assaultive toward those who seek to help them, and this would include themselves. Whoever they are, some of these individuals see cognitive interventions as undercutting their sadomasochistic protective shell. Many therapists recognize that cognitive therapy by definition assigns people a measure of responsibility for their own troubles. As a result, they see the therapist's interpretations as attacks, much as paranoid people see reasonable questions even about things pertinent to their own interests as assaultive and accusatory ("You are not asking questions of me, you are questioning me"). Thus, you ask a person who hires you about his insurance coverage, and he or she takes that as an accusation of carelessness on his or her part for not obtaining adequate coverage. So, patients in cognitive therapy feel chastised by a therapist who implies or says they are at fault for their own despair and that of others as the therapist focuses on the central role the patients play in their own presenting illogic, implying that their logic presumably fails to function according to the strict principles of secondary process (logical thinking), and instead primary process illogic (thinking according to the rules of the unconscious) permeates their beliefs, creating havoc all around. Also, as a protective (accusatory) defense such as the protective defense of "it's not me it's you" of paranoia, like any other misguided defense, the logic rapidly breaks down, showing its true colors, and patients quickly become resentful of hearing how central they themselves are to all the goings on around them (e.g., how they are themselves agents provocateurs). They feel, although they do not always admit it, that they are being *warned* not to do something (e.g., not to project self-blame outward and to stop blaming everyone else but themselves for everything happening in their lives). Now, for example, their projective defenses having been undercut, they might react by getting angry and then depressed, develop somatic symptoms such as headaches and so on in the transference, become even angrier than before (this time with the therapist), and having become all around resentful, become inflamed because they believe that those who are trying to help them are in fact siding with the enemy.

Narcissism drives some of their pathological thinking: the mere insertion of a second person's wishes and needs (or other thoughts) into the dyad becomes seen as a selfish act on the part of the first person. "Think of others" becomes an attack for "thinking only of yourself."

In reality, therapists correcting cognitive errors do often appear to be siding with the enemy in struggles between sadomasochists and their victims. It is in fact understandable that mere therapeutic suggestion and at times even therapeutic supportive responses won't help as much as they might because they get seen as coming dangerously close to criticism. One member of a dyad, or part of the larger scheme of things, not surprisingly thinks that those giving critical input of a positive nature and trying to be helpful are in fact being unsupportive and undermining of others—their victims.

But in reality, on balance, as Benjamin says, all members of a sadomasochistic dyad/group can likely benefit from relinquishing their faulty forms of thinking and so give up the anger that is generated by these angry illogical trends, as they give up self-criticisms that lead to criticizing others in a way that turns into wanting others to be perfect too.[1]

In short, punishing and being punished out of an excessive unconscious sense of guilt is too often seen not only as the sadomasochist's natural payback for past but also hopeful permission for further transgressions.

THOUGHT CONTENT AND THOUGHT PROCESS

The cognitive errors themselves consist of errors of thought process and errors of thought content.

In the case of thought process, the observer determines how thoughts stream, that is, are put together, one following the other logically.

Sadomasochists have fewer problems with thought process than they do with thought content, which will be the main focus of that which follows. The beliefs that pleasure = pain and pain = pleasure are personal truisms for the sadomasochist, but although confusion as to what is meant is absent, what is said can at least be understood as making some sort of personal sense for a given patient. When the sadomasochist tells us that similar = the same thing, though we might not agree, at least we can follow what the sadomasochist is trying to convey, and in fact much of the thinking of sadomasochists is comprehensible, that is, the sadomasochist rather than speaking fragmentally (e.g., in mumbo jumbo or in tongues) does not think confusedly. At no point does the thinking become analogous to a word salad, as is typical of some schizophrenic thinking wherein thought is disorganized or otherwise chopped up to the point of being irrational. For example, when asked what he is eating, a hospitalized schizophrenic replies "a bowl of confines," a reply that is only comprehensible if we do a quick translation of what he must be thinking; that is, we have to make sense for him via an impromptu revision.

In the case of thought content, ideation is distortive in a personal way, according to that which is meaningful for the individual (e.g., what the individual is saying or thinking about). In terms of content, much sadomasochistic distortive thinking is the product of the working of defense mechanisms, which are cleanly formulated (e.g., not "I hate him" but "I am a bad person for having so much hate in me," the defense of turning around on the self). Some thoughts and feelings after being dubbed "unacceptable" (e.g., anxious making) become subject to defense counteraction so that the raw (sexual, aggressive) material doesn't come through directly (i.e., in its pure form). Embellishments and simplifications pertain here. Denial and rationalization are rife in this form of thinking. Sadomasochists deny or can't remember a seduction or, in masochistic fashion, convince themselves that it is they who were seduced, not the other way around, or in fact was the other way around. They may be wrong, but at least we can follow what they are saying.

Furthermore, there is an intimate relationship between thought content and feeling/mood. To some extent an affective component routinely contaminates the thinking content and process, and further exploration reveals a deep connection of sadomasochistic thought to affective disorder, depression in particular. A careful exploration of sadomasochistic thought indicates that a brief affective splurge precedes each sadomasochistic thoughtful production. As one would expect, anger and love are the two basic emotions generally involved in creating distortive ideation, in particular of content. Depressed sadomasochistic thinkers, for example, are generally consumed by the fate of the world and what to do about it, more than anything else. Furthermore, we can understand what they mean to convey. It is unlikely that they would refer to the world as a bowl of confines (that would be a process disorder). Social issues, of course, influence feeling and hence thought content.

The motivation for sadomasochists to permit distortive content thinking is difficult to comprehend, even disturbing. Why would anyone want to think in any way but correctly? Why wouldn't we all want to keep our thoughts absolutely plastered to reality to learn what is actually going on inside and in the real world and how one merges with the other?

Continuing in the realm of exploring content, sadomasochists can be especially attuned by a need for self-expression, but they fail to assay the consequences of what they think about as well as the consequences of what they say and do, which involves inducing punishment or eliciting permission, obtaining inner composure or agitating themselves or others, influencing other's opinion/behavior accurately or turning it into the opposite of rational, being supportive or divisive, thinking depending on the prevailing winds of Eros versus Thanatos, and whether what they say encourages others to interact with the sadomasochist or ignores them now or in future times. They deliberately, if unconsciously, forget that people who are not hard masochists don't necessarily enjoy being abused by someone who gets paranoid every time you ask them a simple question. These days they send e-mails that inaccurately convey what they mean because things such as emotions conveyed by hard text can't be easily included in such communications.

Also in terms of content, sadomasochists generally fail to distinguish imagination from reality as they get riled up about unimportant things that exist mainly in their mind. This often happens when anger takes over to the point that sadomasochists cannot (and don't care to) differentiate right (justified) from wrong (imagined). Painful emotions of a sexual and aggressive nature are constantly having to be dealt with. Managing such feelings involves scrubbing them clean, often via the use of defenses whose goal ought to be improving one's mental health, not finding ways to modify thought for the purpose of excusing the hurting of oneself or others as they accentuate the negative to produce a hurtful effect on the listener.

Thought content can be generated biologically (e.g., via the induction of pain) or emotionally (e.g., via shifting identifications with various social groups and political subdivisions). Put-downs (humiliations of others) are essential to giving sadomasochists fuel for their fire. Sadomasochists distort their identity as haters or lovers in order to project an image they care to set forth, one that reflects rebellion or submission. Martyrdom or rebellion or an admixture of both are found whose purpose is to submit to or confront a rival. Too frequently, a process of retrospective distortion takes over as purported past resentments surface due to situational events in the here and now reviving incorrect recall of past events.

Cognitive errors of content are not always negative and disruptive. Many are made in the service of getting along with other people. Too many sadomasochists find themselves humiliated for being outcasts, while many other masochists are tied into a group where congratulations for fitting in, not maintaining one's principles in a solitary fashion, is what satisfies.

Cognitive errors of content are often installed so that one looks good and is socially validated. As an example, the pocket protector is in fact a good idea because it gets the job done. But these days masochists prefer to scar their shirt rather than protect their pockets. They do so out of a fear that they will be humiliated, so we no longer see pocket protectors because masochists fear that they will be punished for looking ridiculous. They suffer for a good principle, one that is not inherently misguided.

Once a patient borrowed a briefcase from his aunt; the briefcase's handles were covered by soft felt sewn on as a ring around the handles, intended to protect the skin of the hands from being rubbed. And the other kids in the classroom never let him forget how precious/fey that looked. The kids beat up on him verbally, unmercifully, for being unstylish, or worse. Such kids belonged to a group that didn't worry about getting the job done, only about how one looked in their crowd while doing it. What got the job done didn't matter as much to them as what polished one's appearance. The carrier of the briefcase continued to self-punish and bring himself down in order to please the group, his superego determinant. Ultimately group psychopathology seemed to demand action from him (take off the felt), then action accomplished, they gave him a gold star that was of no particular use for him because it had no actual real value, only a symbolic value, that pertained as he now projected a desirable image no matter how in real life the image counted for more than the process—sparing the skin from being rubbed off the fingers.

In such situations of ongoing conflict, no work of any real value gets done; when it comes to image, one is pleased with oneself but attains nothing worth having or keeping except for bragging rights that impress oneself as much as it makes one look foolish to others. Self-sacrifice prevails over the wish not to be an outcast: to be accepted into a fraternity where they could potentially get ahead and find themselves socially validated by their small in-group at the expense of being stalled in real life, to be accepted into the brotherhood/fraternity only to find that the only real reward for rubbing off one's skin is limited to superficial and transient camaraderie.

What works theoretically becomes less important than the quality of relationships. But acceptance isn't forthcoming anyway, because others are talking behind their back, still hazing them but now even more surreptitiously. Masochists will do anything to be accepted; sadists will do anything to make certain that others feel unacceptable.

In terms of specific content, fears of damage and abandonment abound. The sadistic superego needs to punish and the masochistic ego needs to be punished out of an excessive unconscious sense of guilt, with the pain being both payment for past and permission for further transgressions. The mastery implied in a successful search for perfectionism leads to stalemate or other special forms of suffering.

Overall, cognition content represents guilty preoccupation. A favored preoccupation topic seems to be punishment in hindsight for forbidden unacceptable oedipal desires and the oedipal aggression this once implied.

Guilt forces lead both to self-destructive behavior and retaliation toward others who presumably have made one feel guilty or are initiating their most horrific fantasies.

The goal of sadomasochistic content now becomes retaliation involving making oneself/others feel guilty in their deserved or undeserved turn, enhancing punishment instead of fostering creativity, with moving on as a process never given first priority as one struggles, defying Santayana,[2] should understanding the past be to no avail or make matters worse.

SPECIFIC ERRONEOUS BELIEFS

The following are some specific erroneous beliefs that set people into a sadomasochistic rage/frenzy at themselves, at others, or both.

The erroneous belief that it's better to be safe than sorry (i.e., that holding yourself back as safe bests taking a chance on the possibility that one can be even more productive if one isn't so conservative). Safety is a good thing because it avoids conflict with certain persons. Therefore, one thinks that per se the thing to do is to back off lest one put oneself in danger with one's peers, seeming to stand apart from and outdoing others in his or her crowd. The hope is that self-punishment and bringing oneself down, squelching one's talent in order to reestablish the parity that one's superego seems to demand, facilitates not falling behind but instead advancement. But holding oneself back mostly leads to masochistic self-destructive behavior and never works out as retaliation toward others who are perceived as one's betters.

The erroneous belief that one's needs, just because they are meaningful and significant, are thereby excessive or inappropriate and so should be downplayed/modified/hidden or abandoned. Some sadomasochists feel themselves humiliated for being needy in any respect. This self-attitude is likely to generate features of a passive-dependent personality disorder as the individual stays in the shadows for fear of being hurt, criticized, or abandoned if he or she speaks up about what he or she does or should want. (Mostly deprivation if it lasts long enough or is potent enough turns to escalating protective self-devaluation and even destructive anger at one's victims for putting one down.)

The erroneous belief that similar things are the same thing. Sadomasochists try to excuse/rationalize their actions by citing differences between what they thought and did and something else, whereas in fact the differences are too insubstantial to be meaningful, and the individuals involved should leave a little more room for constructive discussion.

The erroneous belief that the part = the whole. This example of a cognitive error that sadomasochists commonly make involves false equivalent thinking such as the belief that having any character disorder usurps one's identity, so as a result one's functioning is fatally affected overall. The belief is that imperfect = no good at all. This is behind the belief that one ought to be punished for one's imperfections, for which one's entire personality is the subject and object. First, psychopathology, like narcissism, may not affect one's ability to function in a global way, and second, one's psychopathology, like narcissism, may actually enhance one's functioning. Sadomasochists might condemn narcissism as per se a quality of defective leadership and narcissists for being bad leaders just on that quality alone, but self-love can actually enhance their ability to lead. Many aspects of a specific personality disorder including masochism itself can be overlooked/ignored, and many aspects of most any given character disorder can be buried in the good positive aspects of one's character functioning. The rebelliousness of reverse chic can and often does enhance creativity. Being able and willing to defeat and even despise a rival may for some be considered an asset (motivation), not a character flaw. A degree of vengefulness in the microcosm is often a motivator/setting for one's good actions in the macrocosm.

In today's political climate, sadomasochists demand of their leaders full participation to the bottom of a healthy identity. For example, socioculturally speaking, the belief that imperfect = no good at all produces the wish to punish certain political figures in the public life for their imperfections in their private functioning. Trivial or important personal issues become the entire measure of one's political ability. Though the brain is divided into separate segments, each with different functions, one considers the brain as an irreducible whole when evaluating the person, valuating him or her in his or her entirety. Thus, if a leader suffers from narcissistic personality disorder or cyclothymic personality disorder, it is taken to mean that he or she cannot function as a highly placed leader of men and women in *any* venue. Additionally, the protective and creative aspects of narcissism are overlooked/ignored and forgotten. The character disorder can be overridden/bypassed when it comes to professional functioning, the individuals in question so willing.

One's full identity consists of a number of parts (factors), and one can be properly arrayed for a job without having them all line up as 100 percent favorable. The eternal question exists without a good answer in my opinion: should Wagner's music be trashed because Wagner was by some considered to be an anti-Semite? All protective and creative aspects involving narcissism should not be, but too often are, overlooked/ignored in the realization that specialized parts of the brain are active in creating/defining the person as a whole. Where, for example, do the frontal lobes fit into the picture? What about the patient who was unable to remember the name of a piece of music he heard on the radio but was able to hum the entire piece through nevertheless? What is to be done with the great conductor who is also a shoplifter? Is it sadistic to fire him immediately, or is there a way to continue to reap the benefits of his talent without condoning the negative aspects of his behavior as a whole? In other words, to what extent should our own sadomasochism be selective as we evaluate people and try to treat them not in a hurtful way but instead in a humanitarian, even forgiving and creative, fashion overall?

The erroneous belief that full perfection is the prerequisite of adequate functioning belongs here. Sadomasochists as the prerequisite for adequate functioning demand full and complete participation in the philosophy that imperfect = no good at all, producing the wish to punish others not only for their big failures but also for their little failures. Sadomasochists forget that those who lead are often doing so effectively only because they accept imperfections *in themselves* and are therefore relatively immune to criticism from others, which they expect to get and seem to not mind getting.

In particular, sadomasochists' "some = all" thinking demands full selection and full consideration of one or another's misdeeds. A typical double bind that sadomasochists put others in is to ask others to evaluate a piece of work they did honestly, then become upset when anything at all critical is said about it, as if the whole work is defective, not just one aspect of it.

Or, for example, socioculturally speaking, there is the belief that imperfect = no good at all, which leads to the wish to punish certain political figures just for their personal imperfections as if they must necessarily be interferences with their professional functioning. Deviations, so often trivial personal issues, become the (ad hominem) measure of a leader's professional qualifications/functional ability. A personality disorder is confused with a psychosis even when negative feedback leads to positive adjustments. One's full capacity, including one's identity, consists of a number of parts (factors), and one can be suited for a given job without having their identities all line up as 100 percent favorable for that particular venue/profession. There is not necessarily significant overlap between "who I am" and "how well I function in specific areas of my life" both as a person and as a professional. Indeed, the true sadomasochist is often one whose rebelliousness makes for a leader who gets things done in spite of his or her character flaws. Political acumen comes from a basically different part of the mind than sexuality, where only certain functional gaps make for problems with functionality. One can congratulate oneself for a job well done even though one has only done it spottily.

Social "repairs" that are in fact socially destructive are often inspired by such beliefs and are seriously disruptive when one awards a gold star to some that makes others feel seriously deprived and hurtfully attacked for only being bronze.

The erroneous belief that imperfect = no good at all, an idea generally found in those with an obsessional bent, is based on a need for complete goodness, with any deviation from one's own personal ideals forbidden because it acts as a universally destructive contaminant. Hence, sadomasochists sensitive to imperfection generally view themselves as dirty and view others in the same light and punish those who don't fully "clean up their act." The idea is rife in politics, where a president must be superhuman to function effectively. Crews's[3] book on Sigmund Freud reports the apparently shamefaced fact that he masturbated and was likely to have experienced diminished potency during marriage and implies that this is a black mark on his character and perhaps even a reason for discarding his insights. Sadomasochists find rationalizations in segmental thinking whereby the part = the whole. Thus, the wish to punish certain people in power comes out of the "disgusting" recognition that they were and are all too human, especially about matters of sex where certain sexual improprieties are considered reason enough to throw a person's entire valid endeavors out. The protective and creative aspects of sadomasochism and narcissism (e.g., the willingness to fight when provoked) are also overlooked/ignored, and that the character disorder can be overridden/bypassed is not considered as central/significant. To avoid being taken down by sadomasochists, it then becomes necessary to project a certain image that is often at odds with an image that reflects who one really is and actually gets something useful done—besides self-punishment and bringing oneself and others down in order to reestablish the uniformity that others' superego seems to demand of other people.

The erroneous belief that reverse chic = an asset and fitting in = a liability. Many sadomasochists feel that it is a good idea to advocate reverse chic for themselves and others as a way to *épater le bourgeois,* though it only hurts their chances of getting ahead in a real world where success and accomplishment do not involve congratulating oneself for doing the reverse of what the culture and hence the job requires/demands. Sadomasochists forget that life on the Internet is prolonged or forever, and reverse chic philosophies in action don't always look good on one's resume 10 years later.

The erroneous belief that guilt whatever the source and reason is a good thing. Primarily but not exclusively, sadomasochism is related to guilty thinking and so is profitably viewed as the outcome of having guilty thoughts, which are then being put into action. Primarily, psychoanalysis sees the pain and suffering of masochism as punishment for forbidden unacceptable oedipal desires and aggressions. Self-punishment is installed to mollify or entirely avoid the perception or actuality of the danger of retaliation and thus damage to oneself and abandonment. Once again, the sadistic superego needs to punish and the masochistic ego needs to be punished out of an excessive and often unconscious sense of guilt, with the pain both payment for past and permission for further transgressions.

Sadomasochists are, however, not always entirely unaware that their guilt feelings are unrealistic; many know that they are, but they act as if they are properly obsessed by having to avoid some particular joyful aspect of life and can't stop thinking negatively as they do and so must behave. At times, these subtle self-defeating guilty cognitions creep into functionality and guide one astray to the extent that the belief systems of sadomasochistic patients have become so corrupt (intrusive) that the thoughts that produce individual guilt (suggesting masochistic self-punishment, rage at others telling themselves to punish themselves, and punishing others harshly) are so organized and centralized that guilt forces lead both to major self-destructive behavior and retaliation toward others who have presumably provoked one to feel guilty. At times, the problem becomes so severe that guilty preoccupations that pertain and often prevail in individuals who are sadomasochistic not only take over one's belief systems completely but also lead to the formation of social anti-injustice groups that deal with individual guilt by forming bands of like-minded (punitive) civilians to utilize the power of numbers enlisting, turning individual guilt into movements to overturn social injustice so that there will supposedly no longer be anything for anyone to be guilty about. The next step is to take one's guilt-driven show on the road by forming protest groups where "I am bad" becomes "you are bad, like me, and have to change for me and the fate of the world." What has happened is that the sadomasochist's chosen libidinal and anger styles are so fused that they have become partially if not completely not only cognitively misguided but also, practically speaking, excessively influential. For example, there is a close relationship between some = all thinking and anger over oneself and others for being imperfect expressed in the sadomasochistic anger style of "if you are not all good, e.g., if you are at all flawed, you are no good at all," creating excessive perfectionism deserving of punishment to others if they don't comply. If they don't match up and they work for a boss with specific antagonistic characteristics, they get fired for their insurrections, or if they have such a spouse, it is only inevitable/appropriate that they immediately apply for a divorce.

The erroneous (zero-sum) belief that hurting others is the necessary accompaniment of achievement, so that the individual comes to believe that getting something for oneself per se as a consequence must predictably hurt others and in kind.

The erroneous belief that needing something and getting something ought to be/are per se associated with suffering. Perhaps parents pass on the message that nothing comes easy in this life, for everything is a struggle. The children are repeatedly reminded that they owe their food and clothing, their "home repairs," to their parents' toil and sacrifice. The child is made to feel thankful for every little thing gotten in the past and that they will get in the future. Preferring to be Spartan, however, the child wants to be seen as independent and self-driven, not requiring assistance along every way. If someone gets up to give the child a seat on the subway, the child resents the implied accusation that because infirm he or she desperately needs to sit down.

Social "repairs" that are in fact socially destructive, as exemplified by certain protest marches that demand practice and passion over ultimately worthy performance, are often inspired by the belief that hard work is necessary for worthy accomplishment on every level. This view promotes pseudoaccomplishment whereby sweat and strain become the equivalent of gain, leading to rejection of one's best efforts if they are not painful enough. Sadomasochists like to project an image even if in real life it is only a *reflection* of accomplishment, not real accomplishment itself. Self-deprivation then becomes the order of the day, accompanied by hurting others by depriving them of what they really want, need, and should have.

The erroneous belief/idea that protective and creative aspects are never good by-products of emotional disorder, which is always a bad thing when present. As a result, the emotional problems that most of us have are automatically condemned, and the masochist condemns him or herself as deficient and does a damning life search about what he or she did wrong as a child, going back over and over again to brood about events that occurred 30–40 years ago as if he or she is looking for reasons to be cruel to him/herself now and get depressed, becoming extremely sadistic to him/herself and thus functionally deficient with others.

The erroneous belief that there is a positive moral relationship between suffering and recompense. The equation "I feel good if you make me feel evil" is an idea that goes back to the childhood idea of punishment as cleansing, so that if a child does something bad and is spanked, then it all becomes right again for both the mother and the child. Is spanking a good or a bad thing? This is a false dichotomy, because different children with different temperaments and proclivities (to sadomasochism) see punishment (spanking) differently and so respond to corporeal punishment in different ways. For some children pain is welcome payback for deviancy, so if one pays an emotional, monetary, or physical price, then now one is comfortable and so more entitled to move on and self-forgive and be forgiven by others.

The erroneous belief that thinking should be according to exclusive causes. This belief contributes to feeling provoked when an individual oversimplifies the elements in/aspects of some interpersonal interaction and the other person becomes all no good. The individual able or unable to think of alternatives views others' unacceptable facets as diminishing the value of the whole person and becomes him or herself an unacceptable hater, punitively and antagonistically making one or both participants deficient. (Accommodation to others is the obverse of sadomasochism toward them.)

THERAPY

The focus for every sadomasochistic should be not on "who is doing what to whom?" but on "let's work together to see what needs to be done to improve a given situation." A major approach should involve replacing spite with cooperation and rage with reason, converting anger into good ideas about what to do to not sweat the small stuff and diminish annoyance and replace it with solutions to vexing/annoying problems, a resolution that can potentially exist in most or all given tense interactive situations. For example, a sociopolitical issue in the political sphere involving the Veterans Administration is the argument as to whether to privatize the system or improve it as it currently exists (e.g., as government-run). The solution involves not arguments but rather listing the advantages and disadvantages of each approach to achieve balance created out of incorporating the wisdom and therefore the benefits of each approach into one compromise formation to come up with a good synthesis, with rational psychological reasoning replacing irrational, emotionally driven interactive boiling rage.

Cognitive interventions can deal with anger by correcting cognitive errors that lead to hypersensitive/paranoid thinking that in turn provides substantial energy for attacks on oneself and others. Particularly troublesome is thought involving projecting one's own hostility onto others, thereby seeing nonexistent hostility in others as actually being there and emanating from them so that modest (hostile) provocations that might exist get elaborated and come to amount to too much as things that are likely to be somewhat trivial, if not entirely imagined, take center stage. Freud's formulation "I don't love him, I hate him, no I don't hate him, he hates me"[4] about the relationship between paranoia and homosexuality provides us with a model for the development of cognitive errors that create or irritate warlike relationships if not start worldwide wars that possibly can be mollified/avoided using the techniques of deal making: first getting struggles out into the open, identifying and resolving such distortions of thinking as paranoid re-creations involving projecting by one or both members of a dyad or leaders of a country who would be more fit to lead if only they stopped creating and then triumphing over imaginary adversaries and dropped the sadomasochistic component of their conflicts by emphasizing and softening the role played by *automatic angry thoughts* (reflexively activated belief systems or patterns of belief) in first creating and second reinforcing angry *responses.*

Similarly, relationships are the place to make love, not score points. The focus should be hypersensitivity due to distortive thinking about oneself and others and away from who did what to whom.

In the general arena of feeling excessively and too easily *angered,* sadomasochists have to stop provoking others in a way that hurts their feelings. The most common of these involves focusing on issues of "who provoked whom, and who did it first; you don't treat someone like me this way unless you are only thinking of yourself, and besides, it saddens me to realize that you think that way about me."

Sadomasochistic angry outburst-like responses are also often but should not be based on the following common distortive formulations requiring correction:

- Distortion of the risk-reward ratio, which means that harm and danger are soon to be the end result of any effort, so "watch out," generally for something that as it turns out won't happen anyway or if it does won't amount to much.
- Thinking magically, that is, believing that thought, being omnipotent, can actually be transformed from fantasies/wishes into real-life responses, having been forged into reality as you use your self-awarded magic power to do unto others, to do them real harm. Being unable to distinguish "thinking from doing" and "thinking about" from "having done," as players, sadomasochists routinely equate contemplation with implementation, with the assigning of excessive responsibility to oneself as if transient thoughts on one's part can by themselves cause/account for what are believed to be predictable (but in fact randomly occurring) subsequent events—for example, magical thinking involving thought-action fusion whereby sadomasochists believe that any idea of theirs should be taken seriously and elaborated as if ideation can/will naturally and automatically soon enough become reality, as if one can "murder with wishes."
- Arguing about ambivalences/glasses half full or half empty issues (e.g., which is it, "the lower they go the higher we go" or "the lower they go the more we slam them down further").
- Using emotional reasoning such as letting feelings determine one's ideology and reality absolutely.
- Indulging in dichotomous or absolutistic thinking, which involves an ability to see only two polar (opposite) possibilities, leading among other things to characteristic hostile emotional responses marked by an inability to accept shades of gray, that is, possibilities in between good and bad such as the likelihood that those individuals who are not

all for us are not necessarily totally against us, for there is a true middle ground. This is exemplified by the view that political flip-flopping might in fact be a good thing, representing as it does contemplative holistic uncertainty due to rational conflict: conflict expression that is thoughtful instead of premature conflict resolution, which comes too early in the form of jerry-built contemplation one traverses and then comes to simplistic conclusions that make apparent sense out of something complex. The resultant conflict resolution is misinformed and done just for purposes of cloture, but it is cloture done strictly for itself and in fact brought about too early before a given case is in fact settled.

- Fusing Eros and Thanatos, resulting in ambivalence, as in the expression "you always hurt the one you love the most."
- Being unable to learn anything from the past, discarding its influence entirely to focus fully on the present and therefore perhaps misunderstanding what one's proper responses should be in the here and now.
- Having guilty preoccupations that pertain and often prevail and lead to both self-destructive behavior and retaliation toward others who presumably have made one feel guilty to enhance guilt in others to relieve guilt of one's own.
- Omitting crucial facts/modifiers. A favorite distortion of sadomasochists is to rile people up by eliminating precipitants and instead starting a story somewhere near but not at the beginning, thereby affixing guilt on someone who is actually doing his or her best but now is made to look like the agent provocateur pure and simple, though it is he or she who has been provoked.

We know that many false guilt-soaked cognitions lead both to self-destructive behavior and retaliation toward those others who presumably made one feel guilty. But what is uncertain is whether in a given case sadomasochism is primary or retaliatory, just as if it is uncertain that parental attitudes are carried through from childhood or if current-day attitudes are formed in the present by other nonparental people (e.g., involving extraneous influences), and there is simultaneous retrospective distortion to make these preoccupations seem old rather than new and attributed in retrospect to rather than actually coming from one's parents. Thus, in oedipal rivalry a false memory in those who are currently at odds with their parents, emotions, and feelings, particularly feelings of a sexual and aggressive nature associated with aggressive impulses, emerge now but are seen as having emerged long ago.

Closed (endless) loop thinking is particularly dangerous. Masochism involves self-defeating thought; sadism involves thoughts about defeating another. As a result, sadomasochism generally involves ambivalence so that in an endless loop hurtfulness promotes defensive loving in a masochist, yet defensive loving in a masochist promotes defensive hurting of another, each influencing the other to the point that it becomes difficult to tell when dealing with sadomasochistic dyads who started what and who is going to bring it to a conclusion and how.

Determining motivation can be helpful. Why would anyone want to think in any way but correctly and not emotionally? Why wouldn't we all want to keep our thoughts absolutely free of emotion to learn what is really going on inside that represents a threat to one's cognitive integrity and in the real world as well as in our emotions. Motivation may also consist of eliciting agreement or disagreement, which may be weakly or strongly enthusiastic in a war room–like atmosphere, intended to embrace taking sides/rebellion with the goal of obtaining inner relief or influencing outer opinion/behavior; being supportive to others or being divisive, that is, encouraging others to be discordant among themselves or to be in accord with an authority figure; positively or negatively influencing others by one's actions/inactions; and/or encouraging others to interact with one another without raw hatred.

A couple was invited for dinner; they said they would come but only if politics were not to be discussed. The evening went well until the end, when the host announced that now that dessert and coffee had been served, the focus of attention of all discussion should turn to his elephant in the room, the attitude, personality, and actions of the current president of the United States. The couple reminded the host of their bargain, but his lack-of-empathic response consisted of "We too rarely discuss politics over dinner, but of course WE don't have any trouble with that since our usual group all thinks the same way." The host knew perfectly well that his guests would be mortified, since they were liberal compared to the rest of the people in the room who were decidedly conservative. The guests begged their host not to proceed further with this line of discussion, but their pleas went unheard. They politely thanked the host for dinner and got up and left, but even on their way out of the door the host followed them, continuing to insist that they make their political views known to the group before they left, sweetening the close of the night with an "innocent question": "Who did you vote for?" To date there has been no further contact. Though they were already clearly being provoked, their reaction was one of guilt, as if they were nevertheless to blame for their mind-set, for thinking the way they did and being reluctant to discuss their thoughts as demanded. To this day, they still look at their e-mail inbox to see if the host had written a letter of apology to them. They regret not having handled the matter more judiciously, but in fact there was no better way to have responded. Were they sadomasochistic, or was their host being provocative; that is, was he the sadomasochist in the room?

What was achieved by the following interchange? A hostess needed to have a medical question answered. One of her guests was a doctor, and she knew this, but she chose to ask someone else her medical question "because he works in the file room of the hospital [but is not a physician]." The art of the insult was being practiced, clearly. But why? What was to be gained here? It was unlikely that honest provincialism was the driving force in this case. But what was the problem? Did the hostess envy her guest for having a degree that she coveted? Did she choose to deliberately cause pain? Was there joy in this exchange of seeing her victims squirm, feeling hurt to the quick and helpless to get relief?

Here are some thoughts/behaviors that are generally not considered sadomasochistic but do constitute the need for serious attention/correction, presented under the topic of "reversing sadomasochistic thought."

1. Some religious rituals involving cutting depend upon intent, the idea being that our creator made a mistake and that the normal child's configuration needs improvement over what he or she was when he or she first came out of the womb. While it has a religious basis and an overlapping medical explanation (rationalization?), such ritualistic-like behavior is in fact, according to some, partly at least a symbolic or in fact an actual sadistic castration, a warning as it were of what is going to happen if the child doesn't watch what he does with this organ of his. Drinking the blood released by the process is also thought by some to be a masochistic act for the one in charge. The question remains unanswered: is there a post-traumatic residuum to this interaction (passed from childhood to adulthood and even generation to generation)?

2. The virginity complex. Again, when writing about Freud, Crews, who has almost nothing good to say about Freud, pejoratively (by implication at least) notes throughout that Freud was not likely to have been a virgin when he got married. The wish for virginity in men as well as in women and the partner's wish to be the first one to have sex with a certain person is in some cases part of a moral sadomasochistic complex.

3. Homophobia/racism (sometimes overt, sometimes covert, e.g., by omission). Homophobia has many root causes, but certainly one of them involves a sadistic feeling toward the participants in homosexuality. In the realm of reparative therapy (to cure homosexuality) "therapists" sadistically demand change of one's sexual orientation, though it is pretty well known and accepted that this isn't really possible to any significant extent. The basis of reparative therapy is of course the idea that it is bad to be homosexual, with treatment of homosexuality as if it were a disease, a sadistic attack on those who supposedly deliberately *choose* to be that way. Various rationalizations are given for what is actually a moral injunction disguised along the lines of "it's a hard life being gay," but the really sadistic part of it is identifying homosexuality as a sin and proclaiming that it is a sin to be a sinner.

4. Passing on a sexually transmitted disease knowingly. Here the sadistic wish to make others as ill as one is oneself is often the motivation, as one deliberately sets out to share the pain.

5. Munchausen's. The delusional wish/belief that "I am ill" can be here displaced onto a child's being the one who is medically ill and hence is the one who needs and gets the corrective intervention he or she doesn't require.

6. Infidelity. When infidelity is discovered, it likely is meant to be found out: nothing accidental about it, because generally speaking you can almost always cheat without being exposed unless you actually want to be uncovered. A mysterious entry in a checkbook, one consisting of four stars hiding the true nature of where the funds went (the four obscured letters "YMCA" were not lost on the partner) was in one case one of the more unusual/uncommon signs that the writer didn't want the reader to know who and what the money was spent on. Lying about one's infidelity is extremely sadistic when the victim can't determine it is a lie and invariably is made to look paranoid him or herself due to what are next with conviction called "unjustified suspicions" and knows it is a lie but cannot prove it. How much the attraction to infidelity can be measured by its effects on the other person varies from case to case, but here as elsewhere generally speaking, the victim's reaction is a reliable measure of the victimizer's intent. The sex isn't always the main issue; sometimes it is a matter of vengeance, for infidelity can be provoked by one's spouse's mistreatment of the other by acting out so that both parties are culpable, not just the one who is doing the actual cheating (which always takes two).

7. Advocating for one issue (e.g., advocating for social justice) that turns out to be a way to abuse another, as is true of certain forms of social protest where egoism is behind the screens of proclaimed altruism and empathy. A liberal stance is "help us suffer less, be less cruel"; a conservative stance is "who is going to pay for it?" Sadomasochistic arguments arise out of the clashing of the two irreconcilable positions, and these are never satisfactorily resolved.

8. Moral sadomasochism is based on rigid moralities that are hurtful (e.g., shunning the sinner) or telling the truth about oneself and others when keeping others' secrets (and having been asked to do so) might be a better, kinder approach. Moral sadomasochism can involve using others' social behavior as a Rorschach for one's own fantasies and prejudices.

9. Unilaterally desired divorce and other forms of selfish abandonment.

10. Not answering a reasonable question but instead filibustering (e.g., answering a question with another question, as in "Well, what do you think?").

11. Focusing on issues purely from the point of view of right and wrong. Sadomasochists become mired in issues of right and wrong to the point that they lose sight of one important goal that ought to be functional

achievement, another that ought to be compromise, and a third that ought to be moving on. This may require sidestepping brooding about peripheral issues such as those from the past and not worrying overmuch about important but unknowable issues involving the future and focusing instead on matters having to do with needed resolution in the present. It generally requires giving up certain immediate pleasures ranging from eating a bad diet to adultery (e.g., being fixated on passing treats that distract and disorient). Breaking the sadomasochistic cycle requires thinking about what is important and what is not, assessing all situations according to priorities, and relinquishing ones to see if something in the here and now or in the past can be corrected and the future can be anticipated and favorably influenced, then doing so without bringing up troubles from years ago/the present time as a form of punishment for present behavior or behavior that is anticipated as occurring in the future. The guiding principle here should be "I am not your punching bag."

12. Focusing on the past and the future while ignoring the present leads masochists to feel that they have been sinned against and in response become hurtfully bogged down in resentfully tinged retaliation for happening issues of right and wrong, losing sight of their goals that ought to be simply "being healthfully goal-directed in the here and now." That, however, requires keeping one's eye open to reasonable doable current positive (relational) achievements that make up for what has been previously lost. This requires sidestepping brooding about the past and worrying about the future and instead being especially alert to one's interactions in the here and now. It generally requires giving up certain immediate pleasures and being fixated on how passing explosions distract and disorient from the big picture, which involves breaking the sadomasochistic vicious cycle by instead thinking only about what is important and what is not and assessing all situations according to the priorities of present and future functionality. If something in the past can be corrected retroactively, then do so, but if it can't be corrected, brush it aside and go around it. Also, has a past event such as a sexual seduction been unilateral or bilateral, and has it even ever occurred? Set your goals according to what is really important: not focusing on past life searches and instead firming up relational and occupational achievements in the here and now central to one's current functionality so that developing and maintaining a good, solid, rewarding relationship and a good job come first before spite and retaliation and should be the focus of doable corrective attention if any adjustments are required. Cognitions that interfere with goal direction such as making some = all need to be banished as hurtful and unforgiving and counterproductive defense mechanisms such as denial softened and replaced by useful defenses such as sublimation (by analogy to help define this defense mechanism, "churning butter out of cream").

Don't allow the past to determine your future as you see all people now as a reflection of poisonous introjects from the there and then, leading to your own misguided thoughts and actions in the present. The best approach may be not to understand the past but rather to forget the past entirely (and so not be doomed to repeat it).

13. Psychoanalysis tells us that sadomasochistic personality starts way back in the individual's life; other psychiatrists (practitioners of life psychiatry) disagree and point to the reversibility of old events by present occurrences promising us a brighter present and future.

14. Maximizing the danger one is in. Contributing to this feeling aggressively is the self-protective instinct that fires off when one imagines oneself to be/feels in danger from oral deprivation, anal control, and phallic competition. The response is first merely felt impressionistically and then rationalized as being the only correct one given the circumstances, and the survival instinct is inappropriately called into play in situations where no real danger looms. Moral sadism is rationalized as good, as it takes various forms such as "the importance of getting ahead in a dog-eat-dog world," as in the cognitive decision to go along with the premise of "who will look out for me if I don't look out for myself?"

15. As Christie[5] says, however, aggression on others' part is not always undesirable. As a victim says, "I knew that I loved the danger, loved the feeling of his hands on my throat. That I would not have exchanged that moment for any moment in my life."

16. Pedophilia is an ultimate sadistic act due to its involving as a target a victim who is helpless and certainly going to be physically hurt in a way that affects the individual for the rest of his or her life. Indeed, the helplessness of the victim is part of the attraction, for nothing pleases a (sexual) sadist more than a victim who is literally if not figuratively handcuffed and cannot help him or herself. The argument that pedophilia is morally hurtful as a reason given to not act on one's pedophiliac desires is a true but still simplistic one—a rationalization that fails to take into account the permanent psychological/physical damage here that in fact reflects the pedophile's secret intention to do permanent harm to someone over his or her lifetime.

17. Incest fantasies morphing into the idea that not just incest but all sex is a sin. Moral sadism evolves as a chief reason for putting another person down: one is assuming an air of superiority and giving vent to a desire to be hurtful to others, a desire deemed appropriate but still a rationalization born out of what is in fact initially a pure superego construct. Developmentally sexual sadism may start with physical sadism on the part of the parents, including spanking and sometimes swaddling, which in some ways resembles handcuffing of the adult during sadomasochistic sex, placing him or her in chains tied to the bedposts. Identification with parents

who were grievously nasty to the child promotes spanking for discipline in the adult. To what extent enemas and taking of temperature rectally are acts still practiced is unknown, but to me such actions belong to the triad of circumcision, phallic manipulation (on the part of the mother in the guise of maintaining cleanliness), and anal play such as rectal powdering and giving enemas, all physical actions with a sexual component easily rationalized as being for medical reasons, only to become in fact a form of pleasure for "the sexual good."

18. Misinterpreting a child's mere wish for warm physical contact with the parent as sexual, thus calling it oedipal.

19. The protesting against something bad that really involves embracement of its opposite. However, the fact that altruism is explainable to some extent by understanding it as defensive in no way undercuts the nobility of all altruistic action. The fact that empathy for another so often originates in a projection of one's own sentiments onto this other person (and the pity really reserved for oneself) does not necessarily detract from the basic inherent magnificence of the sentiment in all cases. But the fact that negative sentiments are explained away as defensive does not mean that they are to be belittled. Just the existence of hidden hostility as an explanation of what seems to be a purely positive sentiment does not diminish its value as advancing helpful intentions/understanding.

20. Various rationalizations covering the true raw nature of the anger in sadomasochism, as seen in the anger behind the so-called positive nature of social protest of social groups. One such social rationalization takes the form of pity, which many would agree is under some circumstances to an extent at least partly sublimated sadism. Valuable social effects occur, but they rarely happen without what is being defended against (the anger) showing through. For example, how likely is it to be able to form a certain honest "love thy neighbor" social group with charitable intent without the opposite always peeping through in the form of nasty rivalry with a social group that doesn't embrace these same standards? Hypocrisy is apparent as in "If you preach love, why do you also seem to hate in the way that you preach against?" Antagonism may in fact be the real reason some charitable groups are formed in the first place; then the true purpose is covered up through a series of rationalizations that, if one looks carefully, are patently obviously installed to hide fundamentally "righteous" negativity. At the very least, groups focus attention on the negative aspects of a population almost as if the individual from one group is wallowing in that group's disapproval of the other. In other words, the founding principle of a positive protest group can be "methinks the group doth protest too much."

21. The true motivation of an individual or group can be best discerned if one chooses to make the sometimes "fatal" mistake of pointing out the

nature of the defensiveness. Loving behavior is too often the exact opposite of hating, as seen in how the hostility that erupts will now, with confrontation, become even more available for protest, this time against the person who caught on to and exposed the revealed dynamics of what is happening, and how protest for something is generally associated with (hidden) embracement of negativity toward its opposite. To destroy their subject, sadomasochists exert power on their secret unconscious self. The death wish that exists in all of us must be stimulated, heightened (activated). How do you propose to stimulate this death wish that we all possess? There are communications without contact.[6]

PART 3

Treatment

14

Therapy

Understanding sadomasochism will help us treat not only sadomasochistic individuals but also the society they create and to which they soon come to belong.

By way of introduction, the following factors are important in determining pathology's level/severity and hence mode of therapeutic approach. In other words, treatment should be modified according to Kernberg's (multiple) classifications of the matrix in which the sadomasochism occurs.[1] Kernberg strongly suggests that different sadomasochists have different levels of underlying psychic integration needing different interventions. These are differentiated in part according to the degree to which the sadomasochistic patient is emotionally ill based on such psychodynamic evaluative components as the predominant personality structure of the patient and the predominant structure of the patient's associated illness, if any. There is an important nosological classification, each component of which requires a somewhat different approach. The main choices involve patients who

- are psychotic
- are borderline

- are neurotic
- have a character disorder
- are likely to manifest their sadomasochism primarily in social venues and nowhere else (psychotic, borderline, neurotic/narcissistic, normal)
- lack the depth and maturity of object relations as regards empathy and altruism
- display severe self-directed aggression
- lack mature integration in contrast to infantile rigid or defective superego integration and its healthy (or unhealthy) integration into the personality (the mature superego evaluates, while the immature superego pigeonholes in preparation for determining appropriate punishment)

Special considerations pertain for *borderlines.* For these individuals, the diffuse and pervasive self-destructiveness as part of a generalized expression of primitive aggressive behaviors toward the self and others needs to be observed, as does the degree to which superego functions are relatively limited (a weak/ineffective superego), leading to lack of self-control and failing to avoid acting out (e.g., the patient acts without consideration for others' needs). Empathy needs to be fostered, and severe acting out, a clinical manifestation of the death drive having taken over, needs to be controlled.

Patients with *nonborderline* characterological sadomasochistic pathology but still with serious, perhaps mainly moral, sadomasochism have a punitive superego and can project their punitive superego onto others, including the therapist. As a result, they alternate between periods when they feel attacked and devalued by the therapist and other periods when identification with their own persecutory superego leads to their own sadistic behavior whereby devaluation of the therapist, more than fear of the therapist, dominates. Often under this spell the patient terminates treatment or even commits suicide.

The level that guilt plays in the ability and desire to control one's impulses is significant though variable (e.g., obsessive-compulsive personality disorder [OCPD] versus psychopathy).

We expect a negative therapeutic reaction as an expression of unconscious guilt. This is a regressive superego-oriented defense against any sense that they may be in the process of being helped and freed from excessive masochistic pressures.

Sadomasochism is often diagnosed as a personality disorder according to the *dimensional* viewpoint; this consists of considering the presence or absence of qualities listed below, which can be singular or multiple.

This classification (set of *DSM-5* criteria)[2] would include the presence or absence of the first five qualities only; the last two items below are my additions to the list:

Negative affectivity (i.e., schizoid)

Detachment (i.e., avoidant)

Antagonism (i.e., paranoid)

Disinhibition (i.e., hypomanic)

Psychoticism (i.e., schizotypal)

Lability

Submission versus oppositionalism

Detachment is not generally a characteristic of sadomasochism and sadomasochistic personality disorder—quite the reverse.

Also, the *DSM-5* list of these basic dimensional qualities does not take some of the main qualities of sadomasochistic personality into account, and in some cases the qualities listed are actually inapplicable.[3] This means either that the basic qualities as given in the *DSM-5* are, generally speaking, inadequate to cover the diagnosis of sadomasochism or that sadomasochistic personality disorder doesn't exist (i.e., sadomasochism is not in fact a well-defined personality disorder).[4]

Treatment methods for sadomasochism are implied as follows.

The affectivity can or cannot be negative, for the problem may involve not negativity but rather too much lack thereof, such as excessive lovingness (encroachment). In either case, normothymia (evening out the mood over time) is the goal. Achieving gain occurs through sacrificial pain. Joyless affect is often associated and motivating, a desirable and fostered impediment damping the capacity for joyfulness unless that joyfulness is attained in a roundabout fashion through suffering (e.g., through such negativity of affect/behavior/thought as making certain that life holds no pleasures by setting oneself goals that cannot be met).

Emotional lability may involve others never knowing what comes next, in some ways more sadistic on the part of the subject than giving away in advance what the object can expect and therefore be prepared to handle—the old joke of being sadistic by refusing to abuse (by being nice to) a masochist. Lability is especially characteristic of sadomasochistic borderlines.

Detachment is rarely an issue for those suffering from sadomasochistic personality disorder. On the contrary, there is generally excessive, if pathological, attachment, a continual involvement or at least one that is intermittent especially in the borderline affective state, with its characteristic unpredictability.

Submissiveness perhaps alternating with a tendency to be excessively controlling often exists and is associated with hostility, perseveration, and depressivity. Sadistic detachment where there is excessive need and desire on another's part for attachment can be an operative factor in some personal sadomasochistic social relational situations, along the lines of "what did I do to drive you away?"

Disinhibition can be a factor insofar as behavior is concerned. There may be excessive lack of impulse control, as when one's hostile instincts come to the fore and overwhelm, with relationships characterized by constant fighting. Here the way that the sadist is being sadistic is by offering too much of precisely what a specific masochistic individual wants—the Midas punishment. Here the motivation to hurt may be represented not by a desire to withhold but instead by giving another individual a hard time purposely and directly by killing with kindness. In many cases the sadomasochist first detects what another person wants, then hurts him or her not by withholding it but instead by giving it to the extreme.

Sadomasochists may manifest manipulativeness, deceitfulness, and grandiosity (in relationship to narcissism, where a desire to be "me"—i.e., "who I already am"—disregards another's desire to also remain him or herself). Therefore, the sadism consists of an insensitivity to another's needs to also be his or her own person accompanied by a refusal to give the other person what he or she actually wants and/or needs because "if I do so I myself would feel depleted." An author just wrote a new book; he gave a copy to his friend and asked the friend what he thought of it. His friend finessed the question by answering him "My wife thought it sensible."

Oppositional (rebellious) behaviors become manifest. Now a behavior desirable in itself becomes undesirable through the excessive performing of its opposite, so that we see dangerous risk-taking as the opposite of accountability or see flippancy as the opposite of conscientiousness as representing a discharge of sadistic tendencies. As always, giving the masochist what he or she wants but to excess and knowing he or she shouldn't have much of it at all is one possible way to discharge one's sadistic tendencies on one's object. Enabling an addict by leaving a bottle of pills on the table qualifies.

Psychoticism is to a great extent a function of the cumulative intensity and depth of certain common behaviors. This may be a quantitative matter rather than a qualitative one, although each individual behavior taken is in itself nonpathological. Almost any behavior when too intense and repeated excessively can serve a sadomasochistic function. There are times when sadistic psychoticism takes the form of unusual beliefs/eccentricity whereby cognitive and perceptual dysregulation can convey a lack of conscientiousness when it is a matter of a parody of usual traits/domains effectively conveying sadomasochistic wishes/tendencies to a victim/partner in the form of "goofing on that partner," making fun of his or her legitimate neediness by behaving in a stable manner but here to excess. (One can sadistically make everything into a big joke.)

Variable subimpairments in the following areas also may exist and be manifestly superimposed upon or incorporated into the basic sadomasochistic psychopathological activity and so need to be considered when formulating a diagnosis and treatment plan.

Cognition. May be disturbed, as applicable to the sadomasochist's often autistic/dereistic fantasy life and its enmeshment with that of his or her partner(s). Commonly the sadomasochist develops the false and distortive notion that mine is the only way.

Interpersonal functioning. May be notably dispirited (distancing) or otherwise abnormal. Or it may be perfectly normal outside of the sexual sphere, whereas in the latter case it takes the form of abnormal sexuality reflected in sadomasochistic sexual proclivity (Fromm).[5] Or sadomasochistic proclivity may be reflected in the personality (Reich),[6] and the same may be true of its reflection in social activity. As with most things sadomasochistic, what comes first and what is secondary is debatable (e.g., do I like torn jeans and tattoos because I am a sadomasochist, or am I to be identified as a sadomasochist because I like torn jeans and tattoos?), and it's usually cyclical. Minor impairments are often manifest across a broad range of personal and social situations, leading collectively to major impairment in social, occupational, or other important areas of functioning.

Social considerations apply, rendering the sadomasochistic cultural patterns of one group distinct from the cultural pattern of another, such as the gang culture (sadistic) or the masochistic society (the charitable organization). Therefore, by implication both the following are true: the nature of a society depends on who makes it up and their sadomasochistic predilections, while the nature of the individual depends on the society in which he or she lives and its sadomasochistic predilections. Does society affect the individual or does the individual affect his society, or both, relates to the basic Reich[7] versus Fromm[8] ways of seeing things (theoretically) differently. One's identity ("who I am") is to a great extent influenced by the degree and kind of sadomasochism that prevails in the group to which one belongs, and the group reflects the sadomasochistic attitudes of its members who flock together. There is a common tendency to follow the herd, part of the process of the formation of hate groups.

SELECTING THE RIGHT THERAPIST

Patients and therapists alike are encouraged to select the right therapist for the right reasons in the realization that not all emotional problems make suitable targets for therapy and not all therapists make suitable therapists for sadomasochistic emotional problems. Both knowledge and a thick skin are required for all concerned. Sometimes a patient's masochism guides the choice of therapist right from the start, which is not a good thing. Too often it is masochistic for patients to seek out therapists who will make relational and business decisions for them particularly in the realm of whether or not to get married or to stay together as a couple rather than allowing them, as would be appropriate, to make such decisions for and by themselves.

Having a therapist make realistic decisions for patients represents a misuse of the therapeutic venue, as it might with an undecided couple trying to decide to get married through consultation with a therapist, asking the therapist to tell them what to do, when in fact this ought to be for them an individual decision. Some processes (e.g., the attempt to resolve relational problems of the here and now using a psychoanalytic understanding of the there and then) are misapplications of theory/treatment right from the start, dooming individuals to a couple of years of treatment (or more) that goes nowhere in the guise of resolving an ambivalence that represents personal indecision—making for a search for nailing down a preference, as such not necessarily an entirely suitable focus for therapy. The hope is to prevent years of marital dissatisfaction by doing the right thing from the start, but the reality is that the responsibility should be the couple's own and is being abdicated. This was the case for a couple using a therapeutic process doomed to go nowhere, because from the beginning the problem was one of incompatibility, not one of relational anxiety. In the sphere of solving relational problems, therapists can be most helpful by turning the patients' decision back to them (the patients) and giving them the opportunity to make it between themselves—then offering to help them with the decision-making process.

The reality is, however, that some sadistic therapists advocate excessive severe control over their patients in ways that range from telling them how to think, even philosophically, to telling them what to do, even down to their day-to-day activities—therapeutic sadomasochism in the guise of helpful intervention.

Many patients suspect that a certain therapist is recommending therapy not so much because it is needed but because he or she is filling hours because he or she needs the business. I know of one patient who spent five years in psychoanalysis trying to improve his mental health to the point that it would be appropriate for him to apply to the psychoanalytic institute for training as an analyst, but all the time his analyst never for a moment thought she would recommend him as a candidate, only she waited five years to tell him that: until somebody else came along with the time and money to fill her what otherwise would be empty hours. There are widely known extreme cases of this, such as that of a famous star who came under the thumb of a psychologist who led him around, virtually asking him to totally relinquish his independence in favor of being guided for life by someone who told him what to think and do in lieu of fostering and maintaining a personal creativity that would have flourished if he were only allowed to be his own man. In his case, as in other similar cases, sometimes the best therapy consists of terminating therapy before it starts or at least before it goes on for too long and patients get overly involved in making therapy a substitute for living.

Often patients who accept this form of control are masochists themselves suffering from excessive guilt that prevents them from making their own right decisions and on their own. They wish to get relief from guilt by allowing others to control them along the lines of "don't blame me, it was your idea in the first place." A sadistic element is introduced into therapy should the masochistic individual comply out of self-destructive masochistic passivity along the lines of "you can't help me, and if I have to spend five years proving it, I will do just that"—the masochistic triumph. The masochist rather than the therapist is now back in control via managing the feelings and actions of others, with this time the therapist (and the therapeutic process) being that activity which is the one being mismanaged by being manipulated.

Often a panoply of fears of progress are subdued by entering therapy that is unnecessary and potentially harmful and using bad therapy as an excuse to stay the same. Fears that others won't tolerate someone as they currently exist are too often dealt with by the patient saying to others who are urging change, "I am getting help for that, that's the best I can do."

At times, a fear of losing self-control is also dealt with by abdicating self-control to others—control by a presumably powerful guru. A fear of becoming fragmented (blown apart) by an onslaught of angry feelings from within that might be otherwise taken out on others is often dealt with by concentrating one's feelings and life onto therapy, making one's psychological difficulties, not oneself, the scapegoat for everything that goes on in what one considers to be a misguided life needing change.

FOCUS OF TREATMENT

This said, serious sadomasochism can represent a character trait/disorder that needs to be revised in the direction of health (thus treated). We may need to treat a subjective septic chronic sensation of suffering that appears objectively as a tendency to complain and to enjoy one's complaining while being thankful that one has things to complain about. Also, often needing to be treated are chronic tendencies to self-damage and self-depreciation (moral sadomasochism) based on a philosophy of pessimism and the conviction that nothing will ever work out right. Also, often requiring modification is a compulsion to torture others, which makes the patient suffer no less than the object suffers. Often needing to be brought up short is a masochistic interpersonal hesitancy that not only shows in interpersonal relationships but also can at least be inferred to exist in the inner life of the person, soon to become constricted due not only to a preoccupation with painful inner and external events but also to a need to hurtfully involve oneself with others in the equally painful processes of suffering and allowing oneself to be made to suffer by persons who seem discontented with their lives and conditions and wish to share.

Patients should be helped to get their minds off something that isn't going well and onto the good aspects of their lives, which they may need to expand in reality to fill the void of lack of positivity within themselves and all around them.

Attitudes that originally were attached to specific objects—particularly to one's parents—need to be no longer maintained toward (need to be detached from) these objects as introjected objects as they come alive in the superego and are then extrojected to be attributed to others in the world. The basic belief is that the child is the father of the man and that the "man" is set in his or her ways by the time he/she has reached a few years old. The child via regression in therapy comes alive all over again in the transference, which can be analyzed, that is, called to the child-man's attention; he or she is then asked to become a different person, a new adult after the old one grows up, and to take another shot at life in the adult community of those who are enjoying themselves within the surroundings in which they live and using most or all of the capacities they have. The therapist who works with transference material discovers that what was originally external and then became internalized now again becomes externalized in the (analytic) transference to once again (unfortunately) show up in later relationships with all objects. The therapist should use the transference to identify, in preparation for setting limits on, sadomasochistic behavior in all realms of everyday life, certainly not just the sexual realm.

General principles of insight-oriented therapy apply here; an emphasis might be on torture—of the individual within him or herself and those around him or her.

Because sadomasochism is often too deeply ingrained to be overcome easily, a good first step is for patients to avoid doing irreparable harm to themselves and their work while under its spell and before it and its associated problems are resolved. For example, in the long run, few self-hating sadomasochistic workers regret having resisted the impulse to lose or tear up partially or wholly finished projects due to self-hatred when that self-hatred presumably will simply go away with a minimum of treatment or just with the passage of time. Friends and therapists can help by gently encouraging masochists to be good to themselves—that is, not to respond to everyday setbacks by taking it out on themselves or their work (as did Brahms, who tore up two string quartets that he found defective though Robert Schumann saw them and thought they were perfect). If only a friend were around to stop Samuel Barber from tearing up an early piano concerto that he deemed inferior, one that today we would find so wonderful to have. (An interesting backstory is that of Barber[9] destroying "all" the scores of his Second Symphony, a futile project at the time since I myself had a copy of the printed score in my bookcase as issued by G. Schirmer, one all ready to be performed.) Friends and therapists can help by gently encouraging masochists to at least usher in an as-if trial period during which they are being good to themselves and others, much in the same way that friends and therapists of obsessionals can help by gently encouraging them to be less guilty and more self-accepting, at least on a temporary basis—with new identifications producing, in other words, new, fresh, and more benign introjects (as they simultaneously stay away from malignant old ones)—if only as a test case, that is, on a trial basis. Often this alone is sufficient to stem the self-destructive vicious-circular tide long enough for insight and/or cognitive therapy to have a chance to work before irreparable damage is done to the person and his or her endeavors and surroundings.

Masochists often self-punish because they feel that they aren't up to standards arbitrarily set by someone they know and respect, although not necessarily the right ones set for the right reasons. In this, one-way self-hatred represents conflict with one's ego ideal, and this conflict also often makes a good entry point for doing the needed work of therapy.

METHODS OF TREATMENT

Therapists can help masochistic patients by identifying specific people the patients know who, for their own reasons, abuse them and sabotage their efforts. For some masochists, competitive males make the worst companions and evaluators. Such individuals are often those who bully everyone. Unfortunately, many therapists try to convince their patients that they are imagining the abuse because they themselves are paranoid. The patient ends up thinking that he or she is too sensitive in important arenas of their lives. Rather than acknowledging the seriousness of the abuse and helping their patients deal with it definitively, such therapists contribute to the already desperate situation by denying its reality, thereby themselves bullying the patient even more. Making the patient him or herself responsible for all interpersonal problems in an attempt to foster insight into what is happening and needs to be changed is a common and unfortunate example of this misguided therapeutic approach. The theoretical hypothesis is "you have to admit your participation in things before change is possible." This is, however, a part truth. Masochists are no exception to the rule that one's problems are often self-induced, not simply due to other outside factors such as circumstances over which they have no control and therefore are not in charge of solving. But there is such a thing as bad luck, as a cursory look at dogs in the shelter will convince you immediately.

I have had patients who literally seek out the painful put-downs or buy into ones already there to justify their continued failure, which they unconsciously desire to perpetuate because their masochistic troubles give them the excuse they want and need to be the failure they long to be in work as in life. One's course should be determined based on a desire to succeed, not a fear of failure. Patients should determine what they love to do, not avoid what they are afraid of doing, as when their fear is a fear of loving. Patients should not let a fear of failure be the only factor in determining what they love to do; rather, it should be what appeals to them now, not what held them back then or is so doing at present.

Patients should not seek advice from experts whom they have chosen masochistcally. Patients should seek knowledge everywhere but should seek permission only from themselves to make Plan B their Plan A. Too many patients blame tough luck, or the potential for tough luck, for their difficulties, when the real difficulty is that it is they who are determining their own tough fate.

Understanding sadomasochism will determine not only how we treat masochistic and sadistic individuals but also how we can improve the society they create and to which they belong. Masochism creates social self-defeat in a masochistic society that permits itself to be overrun by sadists acting like Visigoths. Many societies become excessively permissive/liberal not by choice but instead out of guilt for past mistakes or regret over present positive accomplishments, a kind of group survivor guilt, when the best bet would involve forgiving themselves for their past failures, then moving on. (Some, the true liberals, are thus inclined and natively altruistic; others, the false liberals, are in reaction formation and covering sadistic tendencies with defensive masochistic positions, such as dealing with their hatred by being as nice as they can possibly be.)

With masochists, whatever helps gets rejected before they even try it. Help-rejecting complaining involves the subject ostensibly asking for guidance, then pooh-poohing (rejecting) all the forthcoming suggestions (Berne's game of "Why Don't You Yes But" is being played).[10] Treatment is difficult, for these are almost by definition hardened help-rejecting complaining individuals who express this self-defeating attitude by devaluing others, suggestions or advice, deliberately choosing the fork in the road with the "dead end" sign prominently displayed at its beginning.

The therapeutic feedback that makes the most sense can paradoxically make the patient feel most defeated because he or she didn't think of it first or didn't correct the problem on his or her own; even addressing resistance to change can be experienced by both patients and therapists as an unpleasant, unwanted put-down.

Here is one way a friend helped deal with a specific sadomasochistic problem using a behavioral approach:

> At the last "town hall meeting" nurses were concerned that vets who use rollator walkers sit on them and push themselves backwards and then fall out and break their hips. Telling them not to do that doesn't work. Well, I went back to the office and developed a proposal (with reference section) on how to create and implement a token economy system that would involve employee and vet education on using rollators properly and a token system using intermittent reinforcement when vets are seen using the rollators the right way, and if not, they could earn a token by going to a proper use education class. The director has already set up a committee for me to head on this; first meeting toward the end of this week on Friday. I also wrote up a proposal on workplace noise pollution but did not get a response, probably because it might make the VA look bad if employees admitted that their workspace is too noisy to concentrate.

Masochists can hopefully be helped by specifically giving them permission to be good to themselves. Parents can help their children manage their (negative) feelings of low self-esteem and self-destructive impulses in a way that is not pathological. Instead of participating in their acting out by being equally self-destructive, parents ought to help their children find pleasure and pride in their capacities and creativity and develop their ability to give themselves "tokens" for satisfactory management of their depressive self-negativity. They should help their children learn to make distinctions among emotional attacks on their person, rejection, and losses not under their control.

Therapists must use their own (countertransference) feelings about being blamed, tortured, and attacked by the patient to engage the patient and learn about what is giving the patient so much pleasure in situations where there should only be hurt and defeat. Developing self-pride depends on the patient's ability, when under stress, to summon necessary defenses such as projection, denial, disavowal, externalization, and identification. Therapists should not unthinkingly remove defenses (even though these form the body of symptoms) but instead should help their patients keep their useful defenses after coming to see them as necessary strategies to protect a shaky excessively modest self-image from (further) fragmentation. Projection can sometimes be a particularly useful defense as something that leads to the feeling of one's intactness, even though one gets there along distortive "you are to blame, not I" lines.

General therapeutic principles apply to these patients and the therapeutic work being done. For example, many patients' most helpful experience is that of seeing the therapist as a radically different new person listening and responding with comprehension and empathy and helping the patient make a new more functional healthier assessment out of a patient's old neurotic (everything makes me anxious), borderline (everything disorganizes me and strings me out), or psychotic (everything leads to my withdrawal or my becoming dereistic or even to my hearing voices) view of the world. In particular, the therapist should help the patient experience therapy as a process of gaining strength as one's own right to be strong directly rather than by having to gain strength indirectly via the being weak of masochism, that is, via a self-critical relational submission to another, such as one's sadistic husband or wife, whom one pairs with (as if strength rubs off).

Patients should be helped to de-identify with dangerous objects as part of developing a new ego ideal. One approach involved identifying with dangerous and another with unsavory dereistic/shadowy impalpable objects, say those of the spirit world such as the druids or merry tutelaries. Living in the spirit world is too often a self-sacrificial thing to do, since it removes one from the world of reality, hardly helpful to the patient's learning the way to deal with problems that come up in the real world in everyday life.

Suffering that brings one down via increasing self-destructiveness should be reprogrammed toward elevating self-improvement by helping patients tactfully confront their own contributions to their recurrent difficulties. However, overemphasis here will be experienced as blaming, and that will enhance the masochistic defense of "I was never any good at anything and you are just reinforcing that." For masochists, it might be sometimes said that one's fate is often self-induced, and just as in the Freudian world there are no accidents, there are often only deliberate, if unconscious, slipups in the world of the self-destructive masochist.

A focus could be the masochist's paradoxical narcissistic entitlement, which when excessive (due to the belief that one is fundamentally especially deserving but not getting what one desires) leads reactively to the feeling that unless I get what I deserve, I will go on a hunger strike.

Sadomasochistic individuals have a lot of bad habits they have to relinquish. Acting out their rage without first scrubbing it clean may be one of them, for maintenance of healthy object relationships is crucial and important. This might be in selected cases put under direct advisement. Here a possible intent is to help the masochist gratify a measure of his or her aggression in a way that avoids self-destruction, destructiveness toward others, and hence certain retaliation by newly made enemies accompanying the guilt that will likely invade the sadomasochistic outcome. Always to be avoided are sycophantic appeasement and buying love by suffering, a quintessentially masochistic process referred to throughout as "seduction of the aggressor." Also to be avoided are giving out minor insults that prove hurtful and tempt sadists to retaliate. Masochists must think before they speak and be patient with and careful of those who are likely to respond with a rude comment such as "Do you always have to try to run my life for me?" A friend asks me to edit her book and tells me to be brutally honest. Then she sees any criticism even in the form of picking up a typo (she says "going to the move" when she means "going to the movies") as an attack on her and withdraws from the friendship.

Therapists can profitably give their masochistic patients some advice about how to deal with friends when it comes to being too open about oneself. Friends to whom one reveals a confidence who then pass it on are particularly destructive to patients with a tendency to be sadomasochistic themselves. Supermasochistic is telling others of one's negative feelings about a third party knowing that what you just said will get back. This is asking for trouble in a predictably self-destructive way.

Masochists should not throw out hints that worry or alarm sadists such as "we need to chat" without first saying what this is about.

Having false hope is masochistic when it involves assuming that this time things will work out, only asking for trouble with others who have proven in the past that nothing works out with them this or any other time. Masochists too often talk too much, hoping that what they say won't be repeated to others ("You can keep a secret, can't you?"), then feel upset when that turns out to be wrong. Too often masochists complain about a third party telling others something in confidence, only to have their confidences repeated to the person being talked about. (It is said that the definition of insanity is doing the same harmful or ineffective thing over and over again hoping that this time things will turn out right, and of course they don't. The masochist, however, always thinks "But by doing so I might miss the opportunity that after the 10th time, the 11th time is a winner and works out beautifully.") While this is masochistic denial, a truly unrealizable fake hope (a definition of masochism is the behavior of the person who correctly perceives that a disaster in reality is about to occur and then goes ahead with his or her plans anyway or just because), spreading the word this way may be helpful, and there is a saying that if you try and try again you might succeed.

Masochists who fail to take charge of their lives soon learn the hard way to anticipate trouble before it occurs and act accordingly. Revealing only what you want other people to know is sometimes a step in taking charge.

Public humiliation of sadists, though imperfect, can work well if it widely sends the (perhaps political) message "don't treat this person that way because if you do, you will have me to contend with."

Insight-oriented treatment improperly done can make sadomasochism worse. Sadomasochistic patients who learn about their oedipal conflicts may feel not better but may feel sicker, as when finding out that as a child they were theoretically, at least in fantasy, part of an infantile murderous oedipal plot against a rival sibling or a parent of the opposite sex—an insight that may only cause them to feel more guilty, leading to more sadomasochistic responses ultimately on the part of all concerned.

A priority would be for the therapist to use the transference to identify, in preparation for setting limits on, sadomasochistic behavior in everyday life (e.g., "don't do with others what you are doing with me, your therapist"). Bad attitudes that originally were attached to specific objects need to be no longer adequately maintained toward these, the introjected objects, as they come alive in the superego and are projected outward on a day-to-day basis onto the real objects that live in the real world. Similar things (parents and friends) are not necessarily the same thing, although the resemblance may be impressive.

Issues related to sibling rivalry when brought out into the open can also cause the patient to become worse, not better, not along the lines of "I will do better in the future" but rather "I did badly in the past, and now I have to make amends for the rest of my life," so that currently the patient has two problems instead of one: regrets about what he or she did wrong in the past and getting mired in attempts, likely proved to be ineffective, to correct what is happening in the here and now in anticipation of what he or she might do wrong in the future.

If Oedipus is to be analyzed at all, it is helpful to identify and trace its vicissitudes for the purpose of bringing about real change, not merely to show, with a flair, how early oedipal strivings persist into the present but also to show that the oedipal strivings as they started off were not abnormal, that the patient was not a bad child for having had them, and that what gave and perhaps still gives the most difficulty was not the oedipal strivings themselves but rather the parent's self-critical reactions to these strivings. As one therapist put it, in essence "All children want to have incestuous relationships with, and to murder one or both of their parents. So what? This only becomes a problem when parents take these wishes seriously and to heart, react to them excessively, and retaliate by telling the child, 'You are bad,' with the parents thus setting their child up to become their very own (the parents') poisonous introjects."

This said, a developmental analysis should be considered so that regressive elements in a patient's character can be identified and then dealt with psychotherapeutically. Some therapists find it helpful to analyze sadomasochism developmentally precisely so they can see present sadomasochism as a way to suffer to please others now as it was a way to suffer to please one's parents in the past (i.e., it is reflective of a repetition compulsion). Masochistic child-patients as adults tend to bring multiple developmental steps into one relationship. Thus, each single relationship of adult life becomes a hotbed of developmental complexity as patients summarize their past history in one holographic picture (mash) of what it was like for them to be a child and a child growing up, with all early problems revived in adult life glommed together as a compromise formation as a pastiche of having been rejected, controlled, and humiliated in childhood.

The important view for somewhat older sadomasochists is to look ahead and see any actions they do in the here and now as a preparation or practice for relationships in the future. One of the most important decisions that children just graduating from college have to make is what field they are going to go into. Children have to be realistic here and take so many factors into consideration. This is the time for practicality, not romance, and doing what you love is not the definition of getting and keeping a really good job when you grow up.

Dream analysis can be especially helpful for sadomasochistic patients. A composer was asked to speak before a group on his latest work. The night before he had a dream that he was being asked to conduct before the same group, but he did not know how and where to find his wand. The group coalesced into his father, who was booing him and complaining that he should not have been asked to conduct before him, first because he did not know how to conduct and second because his shoes were the wrong color (brown, not black), were the wrong style, had a stain on them, and were covering a malformed foot, "one with a toe cut off, and were big enough to take a bath in." And the father added, setting forth an embryonic version of the trivial nature of what had become standard self-critical material for this particular parent, "Never mix brown with blue, just as you never mix blue with green."

Later the child became a masochistic man who hesitated to display himself in public and preferred instead to keep his "conducting stick" hidden, retreating into the shadows, keeping to himself even if that required stasis in ways that were most certainly not part of going forward successfully in the venue of growing up professionally.

Treatment is difficult, for these are almost by definition help-rejecting complaining individuals who express this self-defeating attitude by rejecting the good suggestions, advice, or whatever assistance others offer, blaming bad luck, insisting that they have been pillars of strength in a world that is too difficult for anyone to successfully navigate (e.g., "Doc, nobody has my difficult background, and few could possibly survive under the circumstances I had to live in during my formative years"). They also project a great deal; while self-blame is one of their problems, blaming others is another because it feels useful for a masochist to be surrounded by a cadre of people all of whom are presumably to blame for the masochist's own bad luck. Stubbornness is a feature of their character. A patient after tripping over a throw rug in her bathroom more than 10 times still refused to remove it because "nobody tells me what to do," the exception being the surgeon providing the aftercare for her broken hip.

Help-rejecting complaining involves the subject ostensibly asking for help, then rejecting all the forthcoming suggestions as they play Berne's game of "Why Don't You Yes But."[11] The usual interpretations that therapists give their patients here can paradoxically make the patient feel misunderstood, invalidated, or threatened. Therefore, it is the resistance to change that needs to be addressed. Along the lines of there is "no such thing as an accident," there are many real bad luck events in an individual's life or at least as many as masochistic patients say there are. Too often with these patient recommendations involving potential change of any sort are experienced ultimately as knuckle rapping for how these individuals defeated themselves. In particular, the therapeutic feedback that makes the most sense can paradoxically make the patient feel the most defeated, along the lines of "this is what you have to do to get better" being misinterpreted as "this is what you did do to get worse." In other words, pointing out the self-defeating element that generally constitutes the core of the masochist's so-called bad luck and even addressing the sadomasochist's universal resistance to change can be experienced by both patients and therapists as a put-down.

Certainly resistance to change needs to be addressed. Too often with these patients, change is experienced ultimately as defeat for individuals who like themselves the way they are in the first place (e.g., those who also suffer from a flagrant "self-defeating personality disorder" of their own making). The therapeutic feedback that in reality is closest to the truth and makes the most sense can paradoxically make the patient feel defeated, and even simply addressing resistance to change can be experienced by both patients and therapists as a hostile personal put-down.

Therapy in part involves learning what the sadomasochistic individual under scrutiny is aware of in terms of his or her motivation. Is the intent to be hurtful, to protect oneself from hurt, or both? Is one protecting others from oneself by hurting oneself, rendering oneself weak and defective? Is one torturing others to ultimately be hurtful toward them and oneself? Perhaps one is being antagonistic to oneself by not caring that one is screwing up just by colliding with one's human shortcomings. Many sadomasochists cannot live comfortably with an unbridled need for success and other perfectionistic goals that drive them to approach unreachable heights, always trying to do better and better but always failing at that, stretching themselves to the point that they can never be pleased with who they are and what they have and have accomplished and instead of always being dissatisfied learning to just make the best of things, especially things that they cannot humanly improve upon. What they need to do is relinquish self-evaluation that is purely achievement-based, the mode of self-esteem determination that is ultimately counterproductive because it resolutely overlooks the centrality of one's humanity. They need to mostly rethink a masculine/feminine ego ideal that depends almost exclusively on being rich and famous, strong in every way as distinct from weak in any respect, always kind rather than cruel, and always passive, not controlling and dominantly assaultive as distinct from being simply appropriately cooperative and rationally submissive. Are they entirely selfish, as distinct from reasonably empathic and altruistic so that they create a harmony between what they need from others and what they feel others must have from them? They can also relinquish a depression that routinely leads to self-punitive behavior and self-abuse if they can't or won't get what they want.

Also, too many sadomasochists need to relinquish excessively low aspirations that result in their expecting too little of themselves, possibly because they are too empathic toward others, too little self-affirmative, and not sufficiently self-supportive. It is an admirable trait to want to give to the world, but masochists so often do so at the expense of giving to themselves out of an ego ideal that says you are good only if you self-efface completely and bad if you think of yourselves too if not mainly.

There are many viable diverse approaches to psychotherapy with sadomasochistic patients. What these have in common are welcoming, encouraging, understanding of the (sadomasochistic) process, the imparting of hope, the relieving of guilt, helping with organizing and restructuring one's schedule/life, and therapeutic/empathic enhancement (of mood of affected others) to bring about calm—to avoid setting off a hair-trigger sadomasochistic emotional response of a paranoid or depressive ilk whereby discharging rage takes priority over being human and productive.

As much as possible, the specific therapeutic approaches taken should be geared precisely to the psychological complexion of the sadomasochistic individual him or herself in treatment. Motivation counts for a great deal, and troubled motivation is often due to a covalent disorder (especially paranoia and depression) marked by triumphant spite and rage. Sadomasochists who are depressed may best respond to approaches that emphasize guilt reduction, while others, particularly psychopathic/hypomanic sadomasochists, may benefit the most from approaches that emphasize the instituting of self-control (superego enhancement), and paranoid sadomasochists respond the best to interpretations along the lines of "You and I don't see things exactly the same way; let's look at our differences," a way to challenge delusional thinking without being unpleasantly and abrasively challenging. Some sadomasochists respond effectively to insight therapy, while others, perhaps those less intellectually oriented, respond better to behavioral (action-oriented) approaches such as token therapy, described above relative to the rollators.

Family Therapy

A problem comes up repeatedly and develops significantly when children have competitive, envious parents who put them down (e.g., castrate them) for being younger and stronger than the parents. It also arises when parents were nonresponsive to a child's needs and nonaffirmative in the face of a child's talents (e.g., when presented with the exceptional child or simply the child who is lovingly focused on something of his or her own such as music, especially something parents have no personal identification with/interest in). Some parents with modest talents want their child to go into a different (e.g., nonmusical) field so as to not compete with the parents. This is not necessarily true for healthier (e.g., noncompetitive) parents, who can be more permissive to the extent that they are not directly involved.

For example, a child crying in the superette, rendering the mother both annoyed and helplessly so, is a paradigm of such a child and, in turn, a paradigm of sadomasochism itself. Certainly children such as this know what they are doing, and one thing they are doing is demanding involvement, and another they are doing is torturing their parents now, early on, setting the stage for a similar act of torturing others later along parallel lines.

Children with supportive parents are not always so lucky either. Liszt, for example, according to legend, developed a severe block when his father died and apparently couldn't get over the loss until another father figure (Paganini) came along and took Liszt under his wing. As with most things, surfeit can be far less damaging than absence.

GOALS OF TREATMENT

An important goal of therapy involves the development and maintenance of adequate self-esteem. Many patients who are masochistic are beset by an excess of low self-esteem. The goal here is to avoid and/or repair (anticipated or actual) intra- and interpersonal injury by asserting some sense of control over one's negative feelings about oneself and often those directed at others as well. This approach serves the purpose of relationship and job maintenance. To paraphrase Shakespeare, "all the world loves a self-lover." One method involves being helped to see the good in oneself often, until now viewed as a mixed bag of good and bad or, as often, as entirely bad. This view, when presented to the world as such, is self-fulfilling.

Self-definition ("this is me, this is who I am, this is my identity," that is, "I am a creative person or an uncreative iconoclastic rebel") has to be rethought and revised both to firm up and when necessary create a new and better self-definition. Even the baby defines himself or herself as a good person or a bad person, firming up his or her identity as a positive ("good baby") or negative ("me bad little boy") in terms of his or her self-construct. This identity may be primary or defensive. Thus, some masochism is a primary self-definition based on what the baby feels about him or herself, and other masochism is a defensive self-devaluation based on what the baby learns as a way of developing and rarely improving one's self-image, the outcome of which starts in childhood and persists until adulthood. A serious component of psychotherapy of the adult consists of assessing one's bad self-image and improving it if it is compromised. A good part of adult masochism consists of self-punishment, which is assessed as being appropriate, and a good part of adult sadism is accepting that others deserve to be punished as tragically inferior and unacceptable human beings based on who and what they are, one source of racism, bigotry, and rivalry without a cause.

Self-Image, Identity, Altruism, and Empathy

Sadomasochism influences one's self-image; it may be self-aggrandizing or self-loathing and depends on whether or not the individual can accept outside influence—that is, the advice of others—without seeing it as being related to others meaning to take over and guide the individual either in helpful or unhelpful ways.

Identity is intimately bound up with personal goals. The masochist may or may not hear others out without allowing them to unduly influence his or her identity in a way that pleases or displeases all concerned. He or she may or may not remain firm about who he or she is and wants to be with or without letting a fragile self-view be unduly/excessively molded or shattered by the opinion of others. Figuratively or literally, it may be a great idea to never read one's reviews.

Walking this back, self-direction, whereby one aspires to fulfill one's personal capacities and without admitting external regulation in to (overly) influence the individual, is masochistic when reactions to others are allowed to become the most relevant factors in one's self-direction. Some sadomasochism consists of caring too much about what others think and allowing them to annoy, frighten, or horrify the sadomasochist even with advice that is good for her or him. It is often pointed out that the sadomasochist is narcissistic. But how narcissistic can it be to always be taking others' opinions to heart? The pinnacle of masochism is always thinking that others know the real skinny when no evidence is present that these others are smarter or more well trained than oneself.

Issues of empathy often prevail and are related to how one views relationships in reciprocal terms. Sometimes sadomasochism consists of too much giving the other individual what he or she wants and expects from us, and sometimes it consists of not giving enough. Masochism involves self-denigration and excessive self-sacrifice. False empathy involves constantly and automatically making being altruistic into a form of drama, doing so for show, with narcissism at its heart, in the sense that the individual wants to be respected as a giver even when the giving clearly involves excessive self-deprivation and is merely to impress others.

Capacity for intimacy is variable and reflects on the individual's ability to form single/multiple close nonpathological relationships with others, which involves viewing relationships in general in reciprocal terms of "it takes two" and viewing others strictly on how they affect one without unrealistic expectations on the parts of all that leave any or all concerned as individuals marooned in their own fantasies. It also involves forming personal relationships that are not motivated alone by the possibility of personal gain, which means being able to identify with the needs of others and being attuned to them as part of a genuine (but limited) interest in others' longings.

In sum, relationships take two, and what is called a good relationship has to be defined in terms of matchup, of which there are several possibilities on different levels.

Society is in turn a conglomerate of personal relationship styles where individuals come together based on similarities of desire and intent to form characteristic groups, the group then influencing if not creating the profile of the individual members of that society. Individuals in turn have a choice of following the society in which they live or splitting off as individuals who don't absolutely reflect the society to which they (one might think) belong perhaps to form subsocieties that live comfortably alongside each other or uncomfortably rebel against the society next in line, one that once or even just prevailed and nurtured them. Societies then as a whole become sadomasochistic if they destroy themselves or thrive but barely and become sadistic of they take over and subjugate the society from which they as a group of individuals has just split.

Sadomasochism not only in the personal but also in the sociopolitical sphere often serves the function of identity self-definition. Attacks on others or groups coalesce one's own self-image via convincing oneself of one's comparative intactness/superiority. One does or does not belong to the S or M team. Appeasing others such as a powerful guru becomes a practice; it develops and retains one's identity as much as does rebelling. (Rebelling too is a way of maintaining one's identity, especially when one is rebelling as part of a group identified by its specific antisocial behavior.) Conversely, individuals with a compromised identity often find it helpful to join a group whose members deny their presumed inferiority, elevating their own self-view via validation by others, though they are as likely as not to have distortive views of who their friends and family are.

The relationship of sadomasochism to gender is discussed often in the literature. Sadomasochism does not = a woman's problem. Feminine sadomasochism has in the past been thought to supposedly differ from masculine sadomasochism and be related, in a fanciful way, to a woman's menstrual events (e.g., "women, unlike men, bleed"). Other like premises are studied, and conclusions are drawn as to how feminine masochism may or may not be intertwined with a woman's role in the family and in society, leading to women more easily being kept down and made passive "in a male-dominated white capitalistic society" by having some identity readily imposed upon them. Christie did say through one of her male characters in a novel written in the 1940s, "When you caught hold of me by the throat and said if I wasn't for you, no one should have me—well—I knew then that I was *your* woman."[12] This is validating but also distortive.

I have had patients who, like Christie's character, enjoy painful put-downs and then buy into them, especially if they are already extant, to justify their continued failure, which after misguided self-assessment they deny/unconsciously desire to perpetuate. If a nasty neighbor is constantly complaining about them, instead of saying "stop it," these masochists make excuses for them (e.g., they rationalize the others' behavior as provoked or perpetuate it because "this neighbor is my kind of person, so I really don't mind; I can see what he or she might be thinking about me, and it's me that ought to change").

Some women and men also justify actual professional failure on the basis of an ill-considered need to please others or on the basis of reality assessment that may consist of an overwhelming need to (properly) make others proud of them to the detriment of their making themselves proud of themselves. For example, they seek success through having money even though they thus obtain it unethically. (In view of how society admires masochistic behavior, it is not surprising that one can thus behave masochistically in order to achieve a desired degree of social kudos.)

Saying "yes" when one means "no" is a serious problem for most masochists and needs to be prohibited strongly and firmly, because it ultimately leads to self-disapproval. It is not much more than a way to please one's parents and their societal transference representatives and to continue to do so even though one is now, or should be now, an independently well-functioning adult with unimpeachable personally derived morals. The resultant aspect of this, the "I will do anything so long as you start loving and continue to love me and don't hurt me" attitude mentioned throughout, is especially devastating to one's healthy growth and development, because it fosters a self-attitude that is ultimately self-defeating.

An important goal of therapy involves helping patients maintain their self-esteem. Masochists have a tendency to disrespect themselves. They deliberately take steps to fail to meet their ego ideal not only in the personal but also in the sociopolitical sphere, preventing or discouraging any possibility for positive self-definition. The operative principle here needs to be: "who I am, what is good about me, shout it out, get others to support it, and me; this is the way I am, get used to or celebrate it."

Developing a group identity through consensual validation supplements and firms up individual identity. The reverse is also the case: misguided groups, especially those with internal strife, leave one with an unfavorable self-image and can enhance one's self-image not for the better but instead for the worse. Therapy here consists of making certain that one joins the right group in the first place or, hoping that things will improve when they don't, signal that all's clear, anticipating that they will make a quick getaway (philosophical switch) if trouble brews.

Maintenance of seriously healthy object relations is a goal of therapy. Here the goal is to help the masochist express (gratify) a measure of his or her aggression in a way that avoids almost certain distancing and retaliation for being a person who distances. Always to be avoided are sycophantic appeasement and buying love by suffering, a quintessentially masochistic process referred to (by the masochist) as "seduction of the aggressor." The maintenance of healthy object relations for the sadomasochist, what might be called a subgoal, is to help the masochist express a measure of his or her aggression in a way that avoids trouble, and certainly trouble in the form of tendencies to self-damage and self-depreciate (moral sadomasochism) as happens in depression, along with a compulsion to torture others, characteristic of paranoia, which ultimately makes the patient suffer no less than the object. Therapists should evaluate masochistic interpersonal hesitancy that shows not only in interpersonal relationships but also in the inner life of the person, both of which soon become constricted due to a preoccupation with painful events past, present, and future.

Insight in the service of reducing guilt is therefore, while not in and of itself enough to elicit a cure, still a valid goal and involves pointing things out to normalize them so that the individual doesn't keep treating him or herself like a bad little child and can get past a self-view that every masochistic has and move on to an "I am only human after all" self-view, one that therefore doesn't require so much self-punishment and recompense for minor offenses. A form of treatment called mindful therapy can help here, as the patient can gradually become aware that he or she is not especially different from the other people in the patient's life or in the whole world.

Unlike those many other forms of therapy that are intentionally meant to be self-enhancing, therapy for sadomasochists should, at least sometimes/partially, be focused on *discouraging* the free expression of aspects of the true self. This is because for the sadomasochistic patient, self-realization often works against self-improvement. Indeed, the reverse pertains for the many sadomasochists who do best with therapists who tell them to keep their negativity inside and display only their more socially acceptable personality aspects; for example, they should as much as possible consider reducing displays of anger and resentment that distract from their basic nobility. (Putting it simply, the therapist may say "Try being nice instead of nasty to people; it will feed back to your being nice to yourself and more acceptable to others.")

As much as possible, the specific therapeutic approaches taken should be geared precisely to the psychological complexion of the sadomasochistic individual him or herself in treatment. Motivation is what counts, and troubled motivation is often due to a covalent disorder such as OCPD, which then might be the focus of therapy.

All approaches that emphasize understanding and improving interpersonal relationships with the goal of helping one feel less lost, alone, and afraid are potentially helpful and may need to be used.

Many sadomasochists do better with a noncritical therapist, one who avoids putting the patient down by emphasizing the more positive elements of the sadomasochistic patient's thoughts and actions. For example, "You are not a bad person; you are just too anxious and afraid, seemingly for your own good, to be any different than what you are now in many or all of your relationships. Let's find ways to reduce your anxiety level by allowing your positivity to come through without agony and reducing your guilt about having been so negative recently."

Too many sadomasochists, having become overly eager to sacrifice togetherness on the altar of the satisfaction of immediate emotional discharge/abreaction of anger, willingly relinquish being loved just in order to be triumphant by allowing themselves to accept and validate all their knee-jerk fanatical rage responses. They should instead gratify their need to remain related by considering altering spontaneous mad rushes/responses due to appropriate concern for what might happen next.

In summary, as a result, for this more than almost any other kind of patient, self-mastery, not self-expression, often involving the conscious installation of self-control, is the royal road to self-improvement, especially in the important realm of the enhancement of their relationships with others.

DEALING WITH SADOMASOCHISTS

Sadomasochists need to learn less self-destructive ways of dealing with sadists. According to Oldham and Morris, they "elicit exploitative behavior by being so powerless and unassertive."[13] They resist feeling guilty about their unhappiness.[14] They cannot continue to encourage sadists to attack them by looking or acting vulnerable (e.g., by indulging in "self-demeaning humor"[15] or any excessive form of mea culpa such as that involved in starting each day out by asking themselves "what did I do wrong yesterday and what will I do wrong tomorrow?"). They have to stand up to sadists such as career-busting bosses who treat them in a demeaning way if only in a manner that involves the boss demeaning them because they do not want to give them a raise. They have to fight back against rivals who try to crush them, such as book reviewers who give their books bad reviews because they, the reviewers, are writing rival books or have a different point of view and against coworkers who otherwise undermine them so that they can get ahead in their stead. They should deal with their sadistic critics not by trying to please them out of a need to get love from a stone but instead either by ignoring them completely or by facing them down directly, perhaps verbally or, better yet, by living well as the best revenge, that is, by succeeding regardless of what others think and also, when possible, succeeding even regardless of what they think themselves, with their negative thoughts at least temporarily suspended as being unreliable to delusional.

Sadomasochistic neighbors have to be put in their place lest such relationships are pursued to the point of escalating and taking over, causing daily suffering that is more suffering than it is worth. I often decry the tendency of neighbors to be unfriendly for no special reason, but as often I think it is a good idea because it keeps you from getting caught up in an ongoing sadomasochistic relationship that only ends when and if somebody moves or has to pack up and go. Sometimes patience is the best approach, as it was with a neighbor who while awaiting the delivery of a new dining set (coming in half a year) put his own old set out in the shared hall, not caring that nobody could get by and that the aesthetics were terrible.

Sadomasochistic neighbors have to be put in their place lest such relationships are pursued to the point of escalating chronicity, causing suffering that here can be on an at-home daily basis. An example is a friend who invited her next door neighbor to dinner, then sprang her complaints about his new air conditioner on him, ambushing him "for desert," and even after he agreed to right the wrong went to the authorities to complain about that wrong without giving him a chance to right it. ("I just can't stand looking at that thing even though it's in the house across the block from me.")

Sometimes the solution to resolving problems with sadomasochist relationships is not so easy. Should racists fight racism directly, or should they simply go around racism proceeding as if it isn't happening, either ignoring or learning from it? Should one respond to negative reviews by having oneself and one's friends inundate the reviewer by expressing points of disagreement vociferously or simply by writing one's next work as if the last review didn't happen, either having learned from the review or acting as if it didn't exist—but certainly not by getting overly involved on a personal level in proving the reviewer wrong.

I often suggest that an effective way to deal with sadists is to become less masochistic oneself. A danger for masochistic workers is that they seek out and/or appease those who hurt them. I have had patients who literally plead for painful put-downs or, should they occur by chance or intent alone, buy into them to justify/ensure their own continued failure, which they unconsciously desire to rationalize only to so perpetuate. For example, they say, "Yes, the life of the composer isn't a really good life for me, so I will go into real estate instead and make plenty of money, and my parents, spouse, and friends will praise me for having a real job and will admire me for having a new expensive house." Saying "yes" when one means "no" becomes a serious problem for such individuals, and instead they should prohibit the doings of most sadists, strongly and firmly.

As Real puts it, "Men who do not turn to face their own pain are too often prone to inflict it on others.[16] As a result, friends, family, and loved ones of sadomasochists are often in the path of sadomasochistic fallout and are usually ill-equipped to handle it. Sadomasochistic men and women impose endless agony on others and should not be allowed to get away with it whenever it is possible to in some way improve things to lessen burdens and enliven spirits all around.

Perhaps they should be more verbal and tell others their deepest fantasies so that others know what they are dealing with. Sometimes the secret involves just speaking up, but too often sadomasochists are less action-prone than they need to be and less verbal than would help their cause.

As Real says, failure to put your foot down can provide a rich medium in which dysfunctionality flourishes and grows—for example, "women who refuse to make reasonable demands on their [sadomasochistic] husbands because they are afraid of being left [wind] up, years later, being left anyway."[17] Permissiveness can cause sadomasochists to escalate to the point that they become intolerable not only to others but also to themselves. Some by getting so guilty afterward become intractable in the sense that overcompensating, they try to compensate victims more than they should. What is necessary for them to do is to develop a clear-minded problem-solving approach to life's problems that deals with emotionality by creating a form of balance whereby there is a compromise between unnecessary despair and excessive self-sacrifice. It is such sadomasochistic solutions that are keeping them from better ways to interact personally and professionally and from solving problems with themselves and others.

Here are things that one patient learned not to do with sadomasochistic men/women:

- He took people who told him to cut it out as being not helpful but instead critical, causing them in response to his getting angry to get more depressed and so antagonistic to him.
- He took others' resentful silence as harsh and passive-aggressive.
- He took others permissiveness as condescending and even as encouraging that which he himself knew he should have discouraged in himself.
- He took validating him as egging him on to do more of the same, however pathological that might be.
- He used all attempts at counseling as an opportunity to play games with his advisers as they fired advice at him, only to have him throw their advice back into their faces with a lot of reasons why it wouldn't work until they were out of ideas and sorts, yet he continued to demand more and better advice.
- He interpreted strictly fears of intimacy/closeness, coupled with a wish to be autonomous and independent as present in avoidant sadomasochistic behaviors, as their prevailing goal, being to antagonize him.
- He wanted to have his needs met without having to ask for that to happen, part of the above-mentioned wish to be passively loved unconditionally and without having to ask to be loved and without his being ambushed.

As a sadomasochist he was in a prison with bars of his own making, unwilling to reach the keys to the lock right outside his door and within his reach.

Giving sadomasochists advice can be full of perils. A friend wants to kill herself and is vocal about it to me. What are my responsibilities here? Everything I say is pooh-poohed; any advice I give is dispatched to the realm of meddling except for her need for help in one area: how to make certain that her ashes and those of her animals are mixed thoroughly together and spread evenly over the ocean. But I am in a profession focused of saving lives, not cleaning up after they are unnecessarily lost. What should I say here? I tried everything, but each reply was met with either silence or a complaint that I was trying to boss her around.

Relaxation emerging from mindfulness (so-what) techniques can sometimes help sadomasochists overcome their various anger responses. As Brandt says speaking of her patients in words applicable without doubt to at least some sadomasochists, "Slow your responses so that you don't simply react to triggers."[18] Sadomasochists are theoretically likely to benefit from this good advice. The sadomasochist boss who fires somebody when he is in a state of vicious panic, then regrets it later, is particularly apt to benefit from advice to conquer his impulsivity/emotions using mindful approaches.

Sadomasochists who think they need enemies often find that the reverse is truer: they need friends, not enemies; supportive interactions, not adversarial vicious interactions; sleeping bags, not punching bags.

Positive replies to what at first look to be negative provocations can often rescue a relationship by keeping it from escalating to become an angry struggle.

Most sadomasochists have conflict-free zones that should be identified and respected lest one thinks of them as sadomasochists all the time, developing an overarching negative view about everything they say and do.

And sadomasochists should always be given the benefit of the doubt. Sadomasochists waxing positively about how wonderful things were in some aspects of their past life may not be issuing a statement of a wish to give up on a new ("you") situation and to return to an old situation but instead could be making a statement of thanks, stressing the positive aspects of his current relationship with you, something that is itself hard for most sadomasochists to do.

Sadomasochists often respond positively to reverse psychology. A common example of a masterful manipulation involving reverse positivity might be the manipulative/reverse psychology of the boss who encouraged his tardy workers to come in on time not by harassing or criticizing them but instead by giving them permission to come in late (but only if *pressing* personal problems arose at the last minute). Now feeling good about the boss, some of the members of his staff, formerly antagonistic to him, became no longer full of enmity arising out of his seeming to act as a martinet who threatened their freedom of movement and their intactness as human beings. Instead of always being late they came in on time just to please him, simply to give him their all, doing so out of a new profound sense of relief that he wasn't coming down hard on them for being difficult, and rather than meting out punishment for their having been bad, he was giving them a reward for their (more lately) having been good, thus interrupting the cycle of sadomasochism and leading the workers to abandon *their* use of sadomasochism as a defensive, self-protective attack on him.

Similarly, when it comes to one-on-one relationships, positive feedback can depressurize the members of a sadomasochistic dyad by using reverse psychology that has the effect of undercutting/depressurizing an antagonistic situation, thereby allowing forward motion of a positive nature.

Blame shifting is also helpful, however transient it may seem to and in fact be supportive. This can be a temporary manipulative expedient for treating anger and the troublesome symptoms that accrue from it. Here those in a sadomasochistic dyad offer to take responsibility for any unfavorable outcome that might occur from misinterpreted sexual approaches/anger, dealing with these things in a mea culpa way and thus somewhat healthfully, especially so because they are dealing with them without acting out. Others interacting with the sadomasochist can say, "Let me worry about that," thereby shunting responsibility onto themselves. By taking the responsibility on their own presumably broader, less sensitive shoulders, a more patient, less overreactive member of a sadomasochistic dyad can be spared having to feel guilty by being allowed (or encouraged) to deny personal culpability/responsibility for any negative outcome of a given interaction, thus avoiding escalation of bad feelings. Put more simply, it is just a way of saying a diffusing "I am sorry."

But like any manipulation, the danger in reverse psychology is that this approach may actually itself lead to a paradoxical response and thus to a worsening of the problem. Potentially, in not a few cases, a member of the dyad, sensing the trickery/coming to learn of the possible truly seditious intent of blame shifting, may respond in a way that is a reverse of the (desirable) reverse response, constituting payback to others as individuals or in the group as group members for acting seditiously—the target's way to say "I am too smart to fall for something so inherently dishonest and even dumb as what you just suggested and put me through."

Problematic Therapy

Some forms of therapy are problematical because sadomasochists, being manipulative, perceive them as such and so perceive them to be excessively and hopelessly trivial. In the realm of the excessively trivial, sadomasochists generally disfavor as possibly ineffective such manipulations as "get a watermelon and think of it as your mother as you hack it up into little pieces." I know of a psychologist who advocates couple therapy involving each member of the couple getting the same self-help book and reading it aloud together, each discussing the other's reactions to what has been written. This therapeutic approach helps some couples, while it puts others off who see it as puerile. For such individuals, seriously intellectually oriented approaches such as those that emphasize cognitive revision tend to hold the most appeal and so stand the best chance of being effective.

Some analysts cross boundaries and get involved sexually with their patients. After a short-term relationship some analysts are truly remorseful and accept full responsibility. These cases are most likely to do well in a rehabilitation program.

Sociocultural Considerations

Societies that self-sacrifice excessively to sustain their moral values as a people cannot succumb to the Visigoths without being bled dry, being destroyed by those who take them over to drain them of the good things they have provided for themselves. Such societies (e.g., the ancient Greeks and Romans) disappear and are never to be heard from again. Therefore, it behooves a society to protect its identity, but few do, sadomasochistically preferring to dissolve under some moral aegis, often one of altruism, just to avoid being labeled as not being sadists and so going under, with the only thing still intact being their self-esteem and moral rectitude. In politics the group that does not vote as a block soon no longer exists as an entity.

Highlights

Most theories of causation of sadomasochism cover the same ground, not getting much further than relating pleasure and pain. The contributing historical figures besides Freud and his three seminal papers, "A Child Is Being Beaten," "Beyond the Pleasure Principle," and "The Economic Problem of Masochism," are the Marquis de Sade, Sacher-Masoch, and Krafft-Ebing, who popularized the phenomena; more modern observers such as Havelock Ellis and Kernberg are well known, and their contributions though limited and revealing cannot seem to get much further than such (questionably correct) hypotheses of Ehrmann as "sadism is being aroused by the act of inflicting pain upon others, and masochism is being aroused while being inflicted with pain."[19] Causality involving the vicissitudes of instinctual derivatives and traumatic factors are universally referred to and generally accepted as being of a provocative nature, while treatment methods seem limited to observing and analyzing the transference, especially correcting transference distortions later in life originating in early deviate relationships with significant others who, now having first been introjected and become one's own, are rerejected into the outside world, creating object distortions that are needing correction if the patient is ever to lead a normal life marked by healthy relationships with healthy people and being relatively free of moral masochism. Also according to Inbar, Ariely, Pizarro, and Gilovich,[20] there is a meaningful connection between guilt and self-punishment. (Occasionally we find something new, as in Civitarese's difficult to understand discussion of the rhythm of pleasure.)[21]

The therapist should always keep in mind that the patient in treatment has a need to defeat the clinician; until this is resolved, therapy goes nowhere. As a matter of fact, many of these patients like it that way: they prefer the status quo over movement, especially movement toward a successful resolution of some of their outstanding problems. As said of the patient who cannot let him or herself succeed, there is an attraction toward failure, so the patient will hide positive achievements from the therapist.

This is to be expected, since masochism is a relational pathology in the sense of relationships between self and object representations and how these are played out in interpersonal relationships. This is one of the reasons that therapists must know how to spot and deal with countertransference problems and not take them seriously (especially personally). As Coen admonishes us, we need to learn about these patients' hating and being hated that arise as we are drawn into sadomasochistic struggles and interpret the material rather than responding to it.[22]

In particular, the transference-countertransference scenario is a repetition of an early experience in the patient's life, when the patient was on the receiving end of painful experiences with a caretaker. This goes beyond the patient's parents and extends to his or her grandparents, especially when the child was brought up with the grandparents. I know this from experience, since I was brought up sharing a bedroom with a psychotic grandmother.

As Markman says,[23] the therapist should work in the here and now to find out about the patient's underlying anxieties as early inevitable traumatizing relationships come alive in the transference/countertransference and the therapist becomes caught up in the drama, particularly in marital dynamics, as we see pathological masochistic surrender in women and a devaluation of the female in men. Especially, as Markman continues,[24] there is a focus on their unconscious motivations: what is the something that the masochistic solution is better than so that the patient can get some distance from the self-induced masochistic suffering as it becomes revived and repeated in the transference to the therapist?

As Margolis says, the therapist should be especially alert to studying deep anger at maternal figures, with cumulative trauma often part of the picture. In this venue, suicidal threats can pull the therapist into being the rescuer and then can lead into significant boundary violations on the part of the therapist.[25]

Notes

INTRODUCTION

1. Harold P. Blum, "Introduction: The Suffering of Sisyphus," in *The Clinical Problem of Masochism,* ed. M. Holtzman and Nancy Kulish (New York: Jason Aronson, 2012), 4.

2. T. Millon, *Disorders of Personality DSM-III, Axis 11* (New York: Wiley, 1981), 50.

3. A. Christie, *Appointment with Death,* Kindle, retrieved April 23, 2019.

4. A. Christie, *The Moving Finger,* Kindle, retrieved April 23, 2019.

CHAPTER 1

1. Robert A. Glick and Donald D. Meyers, eds., *Masochism: Current Psychoanalytic Perspectives* (New York: Taylor and Francis Group, 1988), 1–25.

2. Ibid., 3.

3. Ibid., 11.

4. Ibid., 14.

5. Ibid., 15.

6. Ibid., 4–7.

7. Ibid., 9.

8. H. Markman, "Varieties of Masochistic Experience," in *The Clinical Problem of Masochism,* ed. D. Holtzman and N. Kulish (New York: Jason Aronson, 2012), 133.

9. A. Sugarman, "Masochism in Childhood and Adolescence as a Self-Regulatory Disorder," in *The Clinical Problem of Masochism,* 41.

10. Marvin Margolis, "Analysts Who Have Sexual Relations with Their Patients: The Central Role of Masochism," in *The Clinical Problem of Masochism,* 187.

11. L. Benjamin, *Interpersonal Diagnosis and Treatment of Personality Disorders* (New York: Guilford, 2003), 260.

12. Stuart S. Asch, "A Reevaluation," in *Masochism: Current Psychoanalytic Perspectives,* 105.

13. O. Fenichel, *The Psychoanalytic Theory of Neurosis* (New York: Norton, 1945), 58–59.

14. Ibid., 58.

15. Harold P. Blum, "Masochism and Trauma," in *The Clinical Problem of Masochism,* 145.

16. W. Reich, *Character Analysis* (New York: Orgone Institute Press, 1949), 246.

CHAPTER 2

1. American Psychiatric Association, *Diagnostic and Statistical Manual of Mental Disorders,* 5th ed. (Arlington, VA: American Psychiatric Association, 2013), 685.

2. L. S. Chancer, *Sadomasochism in Everyday Life: The Dynamics of Power and Powerlessness* (New Brunswick, NJ: Rutgers University Press, 1992).

3. Ibid, 40.

4. W. Reich, *Character Analysis* (New York: Orgone Institute Press, 1949). 44.

5. A. Cooper, "The Narcissistic-Masochistic Character," in *Masochism: Current Psychoanalytic Perspectives,* ed. Robert Glick and Donald I. Meyers (New York: Taylor and Francis Group, 2008), 117–138.

6. O. F. Kernberg, "Clinical Dimensions of Masochism," in *Masochism: Current Psychoanalytic Perspectives,* 61–80.

CHAPTER 3

1. American Psychiatric Association, *Diagnostic and Statistical Manual of Mental Disorders,* 5th ed. (Arlington, VA: American Psychiatric Association, 2013), 685–695.

2. W. Reich, *Character Analysis* (New York: Orgone Institute Press, 1949), 218.

3. Ibid., 219.

4. E. Berne, "Rapo," in *Games People Play: The Psychology of Human Relationships* (New York: Grove, 1964), 126–129.

5. G. Stricker, "Passive-Aggressiveness: A Condition Especially Suited to the Psychodynamic Approach," in *Passive-Aggressiveness: Theory and Practice* (New York: Brunner/Mazel, 1983), 5.

CHAPTER 4

1. D. Owen and J. Davidson, "Hubris Syndrome: An Acquired Personality Disorder? A Study of US Presidents and UK Prime Ministers over the Last 100 Years," *Brain* 132, no. 5 (May 2009): 1396–1406, https://academic.oup.com/brain/article/132/5/1396/354862.

2. E. Berne, *Games People Play: The Psychology of Human Relationships* (New York: Grove, 1964), 130–131.

3. L. S. Chancer, *Sadomasochism in Everyday Life: The Dynamics of Power and Powerlessness* (New Brunswick, NJ: Rutgers University Press, 1992), 184.

4. Ibid., 101.

5. W. Reich, *Character Analysis* (New York: Orgone Institute Press, 1949), 44.

6. E. Jones, *The Life and Work of Sigmund Freud* (New York: Basic Books, 1957), 270.

7. P. D. Kramer, *Against Depression* (London: Penguin, 2005), 87.

CHAPTER 5

1. Y. Inbar, D. Ariely, D. Pizarro, and T. Gilovich, "Moral Masochism: On the Connection between Guilt and Self-Punishment," *American Psychological Association* (2012): 14–18.

2. Ron Potter-Efron and Pat Potter-Efron, *Letting Go of Anger* (Oakland, CA: New Harbinger, 1995), 19.

3. John Oldham and Lois Morris, *New Personality Self-Portrait: Why You Think, Work, Love and Act the Way You Do* (New York: Bantam Books, 1995), 365.

4. Ibid, 365.

5. Ibid, 362–365.

CHAPTER 6

1. John Oldham and Lois Morris, *New Personality Self-Portrait: Why You Think, Work, Love and Act the Way You Do* (New York: Bantam Books, 1995), 365.

2. S. V. Cochran and F. E. Rabinowitz, *Men and Depression: Clinical and Empirical Perspectives* (San Diego: Academic Press, 2000), 75.

3. H. Deutsch, *The Psychology of Women: A Psychoanalytic Interpretation,* Vol. 1 (New York: Grune and Stratton, 1944), 296

4. Oldham and Morris, *New Personality Self-Portrait,* 365.

CHAPTER 7

1. O. Fenichel, *The Psychoanalytic Theory of Neurosis* (New York: Norton, 1945), 58–59.

2. Vera Bekes, J. Christopher Perry, and Brian M. Robertson, "Masochism: A Mixed-Method Analysis of Its Development, Psychological Function, and Conceptual Evolution," *Psychoanalytic Review* 104, no. 1 (February 2017): 33.

3. E. Ehrmann, "Sadomasochism according to Freud's Psychosexual Stages of Development Theory," *Culture, Society and Praxis* 4, no. 1 (December 2005): 95.

4. R. Grimwade, "Between the Quills: Schopenhauer and Freud on Sadism and Masochism," *International Journal of Psychoanalysis* 92, no. 1 (2011): 161.

5. O. F. Kernberg, "Clinical Dimensions of Masochism," in *Masochism: Current Psychoanalytic Perspectives,* ed. Robert A. Glick and Donald I. Meyers (New York: Taylor and Francis Group, 2008), 61–80.

6. O. Kernberg, "Clinical Constellations of Masochistic Psychopathology," in *The Clinical Problem of Masochism,* ed. D. Holtzman and N. Kulish (New York: Jason Aronson, 2012), 15–28.

7. T. Leary, personal communication, Boston, October 1965.

8. Kernberg, "Clinical Dimensions of Masochism," 15–27.

9. Robert A. Glick and Donald D. Meyers, eds., *Masochism: Current Psychoanalytic Perspectives,* 18, 61–78.

CHAPTER 8

1. John Oldham and Lois Morris, *New Personality Self-Portrait: Why You Think, Work, Love and Act the Way You Do* (New York: Bantam Books, 1995), 365.

2. Ibid., 319–344.

3. Nursery rhyme poem "Little Girl with a Little Curl."

4. H. Markman, "Varieties of Masochistic Experience: Modes of Analytic Relating," in *The Clinical Problem of Masochism,* ed. D. Holtzman and N. Kulish (New York: Aronson, 2012), 133.

CHAPTER 9

1. A. Cooper, "The Narcissistic-Masochistic Character," in *Masochism: Current Psychoanalytic Perspectives,* ed. Robert Glick and Donald I. Meyers (New York: Taylor and Francis Group, 2008), 117–138.
2. Ibid, 117–138.
3. G. DeBell, personal communication.

CHAPTER 10

1. S. Ferenczi, *Sex in Psycho-Analysis* (New York: Dover, 1956), 68.

CHAPTER 11

1. P. A. Cross and K. Matheson, "Understanding Sadomasochism," *Journal of Homosexuality* 50, nos. 2–3 (2006): 159.
2. A. Ornstein, "Self-Abuse and Suicidality: Clinical Manifestations of Chronic Narcissistic Rage," in *The Clinical Problem of Masochism,* ed. D. Holtzman and N. Kulish (New York: Aronson, 2012), 113–127.
3. S. Barber, "The Monk and His Cat."

CHAPTER 12

1. A. Cooper, "The Narcissistic-Masochistic Character," in *Masochism: Current Psychoanalytic Perspectives,* ed. Robert Glick and Donald I. Meyers (New York: Taylor and Francis Group, 2008), 117–138.
2. Ibid, 117–138.
3. American Psychiatric Association, *Diagnostic and Statistical Manual of Mental Disorders,* 5th ed. (Arlington, VA: American Psychiatric Association, 2013), 655–659.
4. T. Millon, *Disorders of Personality: DSM-III, Axis 11* (New York: Wiley, 1981), 50.

CHAPTER 13

1. L. Benjamin, *Interpersonal Diagnosis and Treatment of Personality Disorders* (New York: Guilford, 2003), 260.
2. T. Real, *I Don't Want to Talk about It: Overcoming the Secret Legacy of Male Depression* (New York: Scribner, 1997), 234.
3. F. Crews, *The Making of an Illusion* (New York: Henry Holt, 2017), 45.

4. Ibid.
5. A. Christie, *The Man in The Brown Suit,* Kindle, retrieved April 22, 2019.
6. A. Christie, *The Pale Horse,* Kindle, retrieved April 22, 2019.

CHAPTER 14

1. O. F. Kernberg, "Clinical Dimensions of Masochism," in *Masochism: Current Psychoanalytic Perspectives,* ed. Robert A. Glick and Donald I. Meyers (New York: Taylor and Francis Group, 2008), 61–80.
2. American Psychiatric Association, *Diagnostic and Statistical Manual of Mental Disorders,* 5th ed. (Arlington, VA: American Psychiatric Association, 2013), 694–697.
3. Ibid, 694–697.
4. Ibid, 694–697.
5. L. S. Chancer, *Sadomasochism in Everyday Life: The Dynamics of Power and Powerlessness* (New Brunswick, NJ: Rutgers University Press, 1992), 40.
6. Ibid., 86–87.
7. Ibid, 86–87.
8. Ibid., 16.
9. S. Barber, "The Monk and His Cat."
10. E. Berne, "Why Don't You—Yes But," in *Games People Play: The Psychology of Human Relationships* (New York: Grove, 1964), 116–122.
11. A. Christie, *After the Flood,* Kindle, April 22, 2019.
12. Ibid.
13. John Oldham and Lois Morris, *New Personality Self-Portrait: Why You Think, Work, Love and Act the Way You Do* (New York: Bantam Books, 1995), 342.
14. Ibid., 344.
15. Ibid., 340–344.
16. T. Real, *I Don't Want to Talk about It: Overcoming the Secret Legacy of Male Depression* (New York: Scribner, 1997), 318.
17. Ibid., 234.
18. A. Brandt, *8 Keys to Eliminating Passive-Aggressiveness* (New York: Norton, 2013), 63.
19. E. Ehrmann, "Sadomasochism according to Freud's Psychosexual Stages of Development Theory," *Culture, Society and Praxis* 4, no. 1 (December 2005): 95.
20. Y. Inbar, D. Pizarro, T. Gilovich, and D. Ariely, "Moral Masochism: On the Connection between Guilt and Self-Punishment," *Emotion* 13, no. 1 (February 2013): 14–18.

21. G. Civitarese, "Masochism and Its Rhythm," *Journal of the American Psychoanalytic Association* 64, no. 5 (2016): 885.

22. S. Coen, "Sadomasochistic Excitement: Character Disorder and Perversion," in *Masochism: Current Psychoanalytic Perspectives,* 43–59.

23. H. Markman, "Varieties of Masochistic Experience: Modes of Analytic Relating," in *The Clinical Problem of Masochism,* ed. D. Holtzman and N. Kulish (New York: Aronson, 2012), 129–144.

24. Ibid., 129–136.

25. Marvin Margolis, "Analysts Who Have Sexual Relations with Their Patients: The Central Role of Masochism," in *The Clinical Problem of Masochism,* 187.

Index

About the Author

Martin Kantor, MD, is a Harvard-trained psychiatrist who studied with the greats, some of whom had been analyzed by Sigmund Freud. Kantor has been in full private practice in Boston and New York City and active in residency training programs at hospitals including Massachusetts General in Boston, Massachusetts, and Beth Israel in New York City. He was the director of residency teaching at St. Vincent's Hospital on Staten Island, New York. Kantor also served as an assistant clinical professor of psychiatry at Mount Sinai Medical School and a clinical assistant professor of psychiatry at the University of Medicine and Dentistry of New Jersey–New Jersey Medical School. Kantor is a full-time author with more than 25 books to his credit, three of which have won literary awards. His works with ABC-CLIO's Praeger imprint include *Now That You're Out: The Challenges and Joys of Living as a Gay Man* (2011), *Homophobia: The State of Sexual Bigotry Today* (2009), *The Essential Guide to Overcoming Avoidant Personality Disorder* (2010), *Obsessive-Compulsive Personality Disorder: Understanding the Overly Rigid, Controlling Person* (2016), and *Passive-Aggression: Understanding the Sufferer, Helping the Victim* (2017).

www.ingramcontent.com/pod-product-compliance
Ingram Content Group UK Ltd.
Pitfield, Milton Keynes, MK11 3LW, UK
UKHW021909150926
475560UK00003B/266